The Student Revolution: A Global Confrontation, 1969

A Presidential Nation, 1975

The Media and the Law, 1976
(with Howard Simons)

The Media and Business, 1979
(with Howard Simons)

*Governing America—An Insider's Report from the
White House and the Cabinet,* 1981

The 1982 Report on Drug Abuse and Alcoholism

AMERICA'S HEALTH CARE REVOLUTION

Who Lives? Who Dies? Who Pays?

JOSEPH A. CALIFANO, JR.

A TOUCHSTONE BOOK
Published by Simon & Schuster Inc.
New York • London • Toronto • Sydney • Tokyo

Touchstone
Simon & Schuster Building
Rockefeller Center
1230 Avenue of the Americas
New York, New York 10020

Copyright © 1986 by Joseph A. Califano, Jr.
First Touchstone Edition, 1989
TOUCHSTONE and colophon are registered trademarks
of Simon & Schuster Inc.
Manufactured in the United States of America

1   3   5   7   9   10   8   6   4   2 Pbk.

Library of Congress Cataloging in Publication data

Califano, Joseph A., 1931–

America's health care revolution : who lives? who
dies? who pays? / Joseph A. Califano, Jr.—1st
Touchstone ed.
p.   cm.—(A Touchstone book)
Bibliography: p.
Includes index.
1. Medical care, Cost of—United States.   2. Medical
care—United States—Cost effectiveness.   I. Title.
[RA410.53.C35   1989]   88-33079
338.4'33621'0973—dc19   CIP

ISBN 0-671-68371-3 Pbk.

Grateful acknowledgment is made to the Brookings Institution for permission
to reprint an excerpt from *The Painful Prescription*, by Henry J. Aaron and
William B. Schwartz. © 1984, The Brookings Institution.

Acknowledgments

This book grows out of the experience of almost a quarter-century of work in and around the health care industry and those who buy its services. There are plenty of statistics and historical sources, but this work fundamentally flows from my head and my gut, my achievements and my mistakes, and what I've learned from hundreds of people in and out of the world of medicine.

I am indebted to so many who helped along the way that their names would fill pages. I'd like to mention a special few.

Robert Bernstein had the faith in the concept of this book to say "Go" and give his support from the first time we discussed it. Peter Osnos was my editor, and this is a better book because of his fine work. Sterling Lord, as always, provided enthusiastic encouragement.

Richard Cotton, Karen Davis, Dr. Donald Fredrickson, Dr. David Hamburg, and Dr. Alvin Tarlov read and commented on an early draft. Several former colleagues in the Department of Health and Human Services provided insights and gathered and verified facts. Walter Maher and Dan Hirshfield helped with the Chrysler chapter. A number of health care industry, senior citizen, and health professional associations and their staffs answered my endless questions and also provided thoughtful suggestions.

Basil Henderson worked with me throughout this effort. His intelligence and meticulous research have been invaluable. Most important, he insisted on probing every assumption and double-checked every fact, and he did it all with great good humor. He is a caring man of many talents and deep compassion, and I've been fortunate to have his assistance for more than a year.

The drafts and redrafts were organized and kept rolling through word processors by Natalie Swit, and I appreciate her painstaking and hard work; that of my unflappable assistant, Barbara Burnett, who keeps my life reasonably on schedule and puts up with my demands, always with a smile; and the patience of Sue Brown, who runs our office in Washington. The word-processing staff at Dewey, Ballantine in Washington was as careful with the first draft as with each that followed.

Finally, I thank my children, and my wife, Hilary, to whom I have dedicated this book. My children, Mark, Joe III, Claudia, Brooke, and Frick, missed some time with me and I missed being with them. My wife gave up many evenings and weekends, always with her wonderful sense of humor, tender love, and that special strength and wisdom that come only to those who understand both suffering and joy. She cares deeply about health issues and has for many years been a member of the board of trustees of Memorial Sloan-Kettering Cancer Center in New York. She has done much for the health of many people. And she has done more for my health than all the doctors, hospitals, machines, medicines, nutritious diets, and proper exercise could ever hope to do.

All of the above and many others helped. But what's on these pages is my responsibility alone.

Joseph A. Califano, Jr.
Washington, D.C.
November 1985

TO HILARY

When I fell in love with her,
I knew how man felt
when he discovered fire.

Contents

maybe reread, if time.

Chapter 1

THE REVOLUTION

A revolution in the American way of health is under way, and it's likely to be as far-reaching as any economic and social upheaval we have known.

The revolution promises to be bruising and bloody. At stake are who gets how much money out of one of America's top three industries, who suffers how much pain how long, and who gets the next available kidney, liver, or heart: in short, who lives and who dies—and who decides.

The revolutionary forces at work are profound. In science, our genius for invention is serving up incredible diagnostic, surgical, and biomedical breakthroughs that blur the lines between life and death and hold the promise of remarkable cures and the threat of unacceptable costs. In demography, the graying of America presents a burgeoning population of elderly citizens who consume the most expensive high-tech medicine and who already strain our capacity to provide adequate medical, nursing-home, and home health care. In law and religion, our judges, ethicists, and moral theologians are confounded by the Pandora's box of medical discoveries that insists they reexamine questions as fundamental as when life begins and ends.

Against the backdrop of these extraordinarily powerful currents, other major forces are moving and shaking the health care system. Fed up with the waste and inefficiency of our health industry, the biggest buyers of health care—governments and corporations—are mounting aggressive efforts to change the way doctors, hospitals, and other providers are used and paid, and to reshape financial incentives that encourage patients to seek unnecessary care. These forces are sparking a sweeping social and cultural shift in how our people view hospitals, doctors, and medical machines, and how individuals see their responsibilities to take care of their own health.

In business, Lee Iacocca, fighting off Chrysler's collapse, was jolted into action by the fact that Blue Cross/Blue Shield was the company's biggest single supplier, that health care was one-tenth the cost of a Chrysler K-Car. To fight rising costs and spur competition, large corporations are embracing health maintenance organizations, which they once derided as socialistic.

In politics, leaders as diverse as President Ronald Reagan—who discovered that Medicare was growing at a faster clip than Social Security—and Senator Edward Kennedy—who realized that even his cradle-to-grave national health plan could not afford to cover the costs of long-term care for the nation's elderly—are pressing for significant changes in our health care system.

Within the medical industry itself, for-profit health care chains are growing rapidly and using spectacular high-tech superstars like artificial-heart surgeon William DeVries to advertise their wares. The billion-dollar merger fever spreading among the nation's large for-profit hospital chains and medical supply companies in 1985 portends the medical mega-empires ahead.

With such potent scientific, demographic, political, and economic forces afoot, the ferment and turmoil throughout the health care industry have reached the high pitch of revolution. Guiding this revolution is a delicate and treacherous business because there's so much of value to preserve. If the American health care colossus has become far too costly and mercenary, the American way of health has been nothing short of miraculous.

The miracles are everywhere to be seen: vaccines that have virtually eliminated most childhood diseases; sanitation systems and pasteurization that have taken the clout out of infectious diseases; the high technology of microsurgery, kidney dialysis, vital-organ transplants, coronary bypasses, plastic surgery, machines that scan the body and the brain and do the work of the heart, test-tube babies, and gene-splitting; pharmaceutical inventions to remedy everything from headaches to depression to hypertension to epilepsy. We have conquered diseases that have killed millions over many centuries, and we have extended life expectancy beyond the wildest predictions of just a generation ago. Our genius for invention in biomedicine and biotechnology promises even greater miracles around every research corner.

We have the most advanced medical technology on this earth, elaborately equipped medical schools, regional cancer centers that are the envy of capitals of the civilized world, an abundance of superb specialists and hospitals.

But the soaring cost of health care threatens to deny even the affluent access to the miracles we have come to expect, and the billions we've spent have not given millions of uninsured Americans basic health care. Medicine's high priests, the doctors, have said once too often, and with an arrogance we no longer accept, that only they know what to prescribe, where to treat us, and how they should be paid. Corporations, unions, governors, mayors, legislatures, every President since Lyndon Johnson—all the institutions our people speak and act through—have had it with the profligacies of the American health care industry. Examples of exorbitance and skewed values are easy to spot. Here are three exposed by the American Association of Retired Persons:

George Rauch, age seventy-five, vacationing in Florida with his wife, Mary, collapsed and was rushed to a high-tech hospital with what turned out to be a ruptured aneurysm. Despite the best efforts of the surgical team, Rauch died less than seven hours after admission. A few days later his widow started receiving bills: $4,500 from the surgeon; $990 from the surgeon's assistant; $1,500 from the anesthesiologist; $15,536.23 from the hospital. Total cost for less than seven hours of unsuccessful emergency surgery: $22,526.23.

Mrs. Opal Burge of Hebron, Indiana, got a 208-page hospital bill for more than $250,000 for the five and a half months her seventy-three-year-old husband, Floyd, spent in an intensive care unit, battling emphysema that killed him. Medicare and private insurance covered all but $14,349 of the bill. The hospital has required her to make up the difference in monthly installments that come from her Social Security checks. Her family physician charged her $800 more than Medicare reimburses.

Donald Funk, sixty-four, of Long Beach, California, suffered a mild heart attack and was rushed by paramedics to the nearest hospital. A few days later, when his condition had stabilized, he sought transfer to the nearby Veterans Administration facility, where he was eligible for free treatment. The hospital flatly refused. Only after much delay, at his wife's insistence and the VA's demand, did the hospital agree to the transfer. But by that time ten days had passed, and the hospital and doctors billed Funk more than $25,000.

As Secretary of Health, Education, and Welfare, I discovered that more than 30 percent of Medicare's multibillion-dollar budget was spent on patients with less than a year to live, usually in high-tech, life-extending, hospital intensive care units, while that same program then denied funds for low-cost, dignified hospice care to relieve the suffering of the terminally ill. Medicare now pays for some hospice care, but most private insurers don't pay for any.

In 1984 Allstate Life Insurance studies revealed to Executive Vice-President Robert Roberts that 30 percent of all medical costs resulted from waste, duplication, fraud, and abuse. In 1985 a study by doctors at the Veterans Administration Medical Center in Long Beach, California, found that the routine X-rays hospitals give each year, at a cost of $1.5 billion, provide almost no information that helps identify the best treatment for patients. Computers have detected hundreds of providers who try to rip off Medicaid and Medicare.

Medical featherbedding abounds. Doctors and dentists perform simple medical procedures that paramedicals and nurses could do at far less cost and just as safely and competently. The medicine men and women provide unnecessary medical services and prescribe drugs patients don't have to take to get well. Hundreds of hospitals admit patients who shouldn't be there and keep those who should too long. Medical equipment companies sell hospitals and doctors expensive equipment they don't need. Lawyers seek extravagant verdicts for alleged medical malpractice and pocket an average of 30 percent, plus expenses, of what the juries they manipulate award.

Such waste and abyse are only symptoms of the peril to the health care system. Eliminating them will save some money, and disciplining abusers may temporarily calm some outraged consumers and citizens. But these actions alone won't cure the disease of costs so high and so detached from medical need or quality of care that they threaten the best of American medicine. The cure requires drastic institutional surgery. The American way of health has been voracious in its pursuit of more and more money, too often unrelated to better care. Unless we change its course, our health care system will break the bank, set off the nastiest generational and political conflict our nation has ever experienced, provide increasingly extravagant first-rate health care to fewer and fewer Americans, and put a life-and-death power in the hands of government, which no free people can tolerate.

The revolutionary forces are already at work, but if we are to emerge with basic changes for the good, we need to be informed, vigilant participants. To determine how to restructure our health care system, we must first understand how we got where we are. Each of us did our share, acting by and large with the finest motives, for the most compassionate of reasons.

Doctors acquired an unnecessarily broad monopoly over the practice of medicine (as they defined it), and we established a payment system that has encouraged them to treat us when we are sick, not to teach us to take care of ourselves. Rather than being institutions of last resort, hospitals became settings of first choice for treating too many minor ailments, especially when the insurance coverage was good. Corporations and unions tilted employee health benefits toward the most expensive care and gave workers little sense of its cost. Private insurers saw themselves as agents of doctors and hospitals rather than of the companies and patients who paid their bills. In enacting government programs to provide health care to senior citizens and poor people, we acceded to demands of hospitals and doctors for reimbursement systems that promoted breakneck inflation in health costs and had virtually no incentives for efficiency. The profit motives of medical equipment manufacturers and the cleverness of our scientists found no sales resistance from hospitals that were reimbursed for whatever price they paid. Our elderly population expanded far beyond projections of just twenty-five years ago and placed unanticipated financial demands on Medicare to provide high-tech medicine; government reacted to its budgetary problems by shifting costs like peas in a shell game rather than working to recast the health care system.

The time has come to alter fundamentally the way we deliver health care to our people, who has access to it, how we pay for it, the way we educate our doctors and protect their turf, the abandon with which we handle our bodies and minds, and the professional and financial incentives we offer doctors, researchers, hospitals, insurers, laboratories, medical equipment suppliers, drug companies, malpractice lawyers—and patients. Most important, we must change the object of our attention from sick care to health care, encourage Americans to keep themselves in far better shape and to stay out of hospitals unless they have no alternative, and give doctors incentives to keep us healthy rather than just treat us when we're ill.

If we don't change the system, prepare to live in an America where the annual health care bill will hit a trillion dollars in the early 1990s and continue to double every six or seven years after that; where the cost of health care makes our automobiles and steel and other products so expensive that American industry can't compete in a global marketplace; and where government rations health care and bureaucrats issue hundreds of pages of regulations that determine who lives and who dies.

It's not a very pleasant future. But that future is now for some people. Whether it will be tomorrow for Americans depends on how we change the American way of health.

There's hope because there's so much variety and freedom in America that, given the right incentives, doctors can compete with each other and with hospitals, and because the pressure on state governments to cut costs may yet open up many medical procedures to trained paramedics.

There's hope because the federal government is trying to get its Medicare act together by offering hospitals and other providers carrots and sticks to be efficient.

There's hope because the genius of American business, determined to compete abroad, is turned on to making our doctors and hospitals more efficient suppliers.

The signals of change are flashing so quickly that the 1980s can become the decade Americans got a handle on health care costs, took charge of their own health, and reshaped our inefficient sick care system into the most efficient health care system in the world. Just look at a few of the flashing lights:

- Health care costs, once projected to nudge $400 billion in 1984, rose at only 9.1 percent and came in at $387 billion. That growth rate was the lowest since 1963.
- Hospital admissions, lengths of stay, and occupancy rates dropped in 1984 and 1985.
- Medicare, once predicted to go bust by the early 1990s, looks solvent until late in that decade.
- Cigarette consumption, both total and per capita, has gone down, and more states and cities passed laws prohibiting smoking in enclosed public places.
- Businesses across America are moving forcefully to cut health care costs and eliminate inefficiencies.

These are only beginnings, and the biggest obstacles lie ahead. I know that from personal experience. I've lived through much of our nation's recent health care history—as President Lyndon Johnson's Special Assistant for Domestic Affairs, through the creation of Medicare and Medicaid and a host of other Great Society programs intended to give the old and the poor access to health care; later, as President Jimmy Carter's Secretary of Health, Education, and Welfare, through many attempts to contain health care costs; through Chrysler's struggle to reduce its health care bill as it fought for survival under Lee Iacocca's leadership; and as attorney for a number of companies, consumers as well as providers of health care and pharmaceuticals. I've watched health care cost increases abate slightly in the face of controls, only to resume their meteoric rise as soon as controls or the threat of them were lifted.

For more than a decade, I was convinced that the job of reining in health care costs was too big for the private sector, that only government could do it, and that government had to do the whole thing. That's why, as Secretary of HEW, I proposed an across-the-board cap on hospital charges that would have controlled payments by all private insurers as well as by the government. My years at HEW, and six more outside government, lead me to believe that the great hope of containing health care costs lies in an aroused private sector. Government has to do its share, get its house in order. But a Congress whose members depend on private contributions for election campaigns, who must satisfy constituencies in their home districts and states, and who will always worry about offending hospital trustees and influential state and local medical societies cannot do the job alone. Our best hope to change the health care system rests in an awakened, competitive world of business purchasers demanding and bargaining for high-quality care from a variety of providers at much lower cost.

My experience leads me to conclude that the outcome of America's health care revolution is by no means clear. The scientific and demographic forces are unprecedented. The moral and ethical questions would test an Aristotle or Aquinas. The human and economic issues are so vexing that many of us who have grappled with them have created problems in our quest for solutions. The health industry players are rich and powerful. Whether we have the staying power and ingenuity to turn the sound and fury of the mid-1980s into lasting structural change for the better remains to be seen.

But whatever happens, the health care industry of tomorrow is going to be unrecognizably different from today's world of medicine. Whether it will be better depends on how we shape the revolution. I believe—and my experiences with Chrysler support my belief—that we have the power to shape it wisely and well. If we do so, we can have the most efficient as well as the most remarkable medical system in the world—and provide top-quality health care to all our people, including millions who do not now have access to such care.

Chapter 2

THE CHRYSLER STORY

On July 14, 1978, I read in the morning paper that Lee Iacocca had been abruptly fired by Henry Ford. The black-and-white photo of Iacocca revealed a hurt so deep that I called him from my office at the Department of Health, Education, and Welfare.

"Lee," I said. "These things have a way of turning out okay. This just *could* be one of the best things that ever happened to you."

One year later, on July 20, 1979, the morning after President Jimmy Carter announced that he had asked for and accepted my resignation as Secretary of Health, Education, and Welfare, my secretary buzzed and said, "Lee Iacocca's on the line." As soon as I said, "Hello," Iacocca blurted out, "Joe. You told me that being fired by Henry Ford could turn out to be one of the best things that ever happened to me. Well, let me tell you this. Being fired by Jimmy Carter *is* the best thing that ever happened to you."

Iacocca's next call came in early 1981. He invited me to join the Chrysler board of directors. I hesitated to accept because I was putting together my own law firm and wanted to devote all my energies to that. I talked to Bob McNamara, my former boss when he was Secretary of Defense, who had worked with Iacocca at Ford. McNamara urged me to join the board, "You'll learn more about business from Lee in a year than from any other businessman in ten," he said, although he warned me, "Chrysler will probably go under. I don't see how he can revive it."

A few weeks later, Iacocca called again. "Meet me in New

York," he said. "I want you on this board; you can really help me and Chrysler. You won't believe our health care costs. Alone, they can sink this ship."

We met for a couple of hours in Iacocca's Waldorf Tower suite, and later had dinner at Romeo Salta's on West 56th Street. Iacocca was aghast at Chrysler's health care costs. "They'll break this goddamn company if we don't do something about them."

I agreed. I had tried unsuccessfully to alert American businesses to the dangers of rising health care costs when I was HEW Secretary. But it was like dropping a grain of sand on a beach. I had no impact. No one heard.

Iacocca was getting me excited about the prospect of joining the Chrysler board. "Look," Iacocca said, "I'll set up a committee. You. Me. Doug Fraser [then president of the United Automobile Workers Union and a Chrysler Board member]. The three of us did more to create this mess than any three people in America. You with those Great Society programs. Fraser with his crazy demands for health care benefits in union contracts. And me—I agreed to damn near every one of them."

I couldn't help smiling.

Then Iacocca threw out the clincher. "You say you want to do something about health care costs. You chair the committee, the health care committee of the board."

I was hooked. No other corporate board had such a committee. And working with Lee Iacocca ever since has been one of the best things that ever happened to me. Iacocca put Red Cross chairman Jerome Holland on the committee, and later former Michigan governor William Milliken and Owens-Illinois chairman and chief executive Robert Lanigan, when they came on the Chrysler board. In 1984, we added Owen Bieber, who succeeded Fraser as president of the United Automobile Workers and joined the board.

We started work almost immediately. What we found was appalling waste and inefficiency that exceeded my worst concerns about the health care system as Secretary of HEW. Iacocca was right. We had a health care cost crisis on our hands. If Chrysler was to successfully defy the *Wall Street Journal's* injunction to "die with dignity" and recover financially, we had to confront it.

Chrysler's bill for health care costs was rising at a greater rate than were any others it was paying. Chrysler's predicament was shared by many other businesses, particularly smokestack industries coping with powerful unions, dwindling productivity, aging, shrinking work forces, and a ballooning number of retirees getting increasingly old and consuming the most expensive care.

Like most large companies with employees represented by the United Automobile Workers and such other big unions as the United Steelworkers, Chrysler had allowed the collective-bargaining process to produce a health care benefit package for everything from coronary bypass surgery to fixing ingrown toenails, with no incentive for its employees to buy prudently. For the big ticket stuff, such as hospitalization, surgery, laboratory and X-ray services, the Chrysler plan paid it all: no deductibles or copayments—a guarantee that employees and retirees and their families would think they had the greatest free lunch since the saloons gave away food with the five-cent beer. To top it off, the number of nonworkers getting these benefits exceeded the number of people still on the job. At one point in 1982, Chrysler was paying health care expenses for 107,000 retirees and individuals who had been laid off, when it had only 61,000 active workers on its payroll. The impact on costs was disastrous. The health care bill was climbing so fast that it was expected to exceed $460 million by 1984.

Chrysler and the UAW didn't cook this stew overnight. It had been simmering for forty years.

It all started, innocently enough, in 1941, when Chrysler agreed with its recently recognized union to set up a group health plan. The initial plan covered only hospitalization, and this only for employees who paid the entire cost through payroll deductions. Back then, no one foresaw that covering only hospital costs might tilt medical services toward the most expensive level of health care. Chrysler was looking in another direction, at the desirability of protecting its workers from the catastrophe of a big hospital bill.

Nothing much changed until 1950, when General Motors, the auto industry's domineering big daddy, agreed to pay half the cost of its employee group coverage and to expand benefits to cover doctors' fees for surgical and many medical services. Chrysler followed the leader. Three years later, Chrysler agreed to set up comparable coverage for retirees, but insisted that they pay the full cost of the program.

In 1961 Chrysler opened its treasury door to hospitals and doctors. Again following the leader, General Motors, Chrysler agreed to pay the full cost of covered hospital, surgical, and medical benefits for employees and their dependents, and half of such costs for retirees and their dependents. In 1964 Chrysler, at that time the company targeted for strike by the UAW if collective bargaining failed, agreed to first-dollar coverage (no deductibles or copayments) for outpatient psychiatric care (to take effect in 1966). The company opened its treasury door wider by agreeing to pay the full cost of health care benefits for retirees and their dependents. It sounded benign and affordable at the time; little did Chrysler realize that years later, health costs for retirees would constitute almost 40 percent of the corporation's health care bill.

If Chrysler had hoped that President Lyndon Johnson's Medicare program would pick up most of the tab for its retirees, the company was sadly mistaken. A pincer movement of UAW early-retirement programs (which swelled the ranks of retirees with members who were under sixty-five and hence ineligible for Medicare) and increases in Medicare deductibles and copayments that Chrysler had agreed to pay sent its health care costs rocketing.

By agreeing to first-dollar coverage, Chrysler increasingly insulated its employees from any sense of what health care cost. In 1967 the company's plans agreed to pay "usual, customary, and reasonable" fees to physicians, essentially the same reimbursement system that helped bring Medicare to the brink of bankruptcy. This gave the doctors the power to write their own checks on the Chrysler account.

With the health care Christmas tree up, Chrysler started hanging expensive ornaments on it. In 1967 a prescription drug program for employees and dependents was added. Initially considered a relatively modest benefit, this ornament cost more than $30 million by 1984, in large measure because company-paid coverage was extended to retirees in 1971.

Next came the dental care ornaments. In 1973 the company agreed to a fee-for-service dental benefit program for active employees. As usual, coverage was extended to retirees during the next round of contract talks, in 1976. Lots of other companies were hanging the same ornaments. Dental fees and costs rose rapidly. Consumers with dental insurance spent more on dental care than those without coverage; the less the individual had to pay under his insurance coverage, the higher the expenditures.

Chrysler hung the final baubles on its health care Christmas tree in 1976: eyeglasses for its active employees; hearing aids for both active and retired workers. Despite signals of imminent financial disaster, Chrysler extended its eyeglasses coverage to retirees in 1979. Once again, these benefits were added at little or no cost to employees. These years of hanging ornaments broke the branches of Chrysler's health care Christmas tree.

The combination of double-digit inflation, 20 percent interest rates, foreign competition, and severe recession in the late 1970s was devastating to America's smokestack industries, as companies laid off thousands of workers, shut down plants, and were merged or bankrupted out of existence. Despite the layoffs and closed plants, many companies remained hostage to the health care industry and its singularly inefficient and wasteful delivery system because contracts required them to continue paying health care costs for extended periods for laid-off employees, and to pay them forever for early retirees. The stinging salt in the economic wound was that health care costs, particularly hospital costs, far outran even the double-digit inflation in the general economy.

The auto companies did make some gestures in the direction of health care cost containment. The 1976 contracts reflected concern about promiscuous hospital utilization. They called for the development of pilot programs, including voluntary second opinions for elective surgery; promotion of less expensive preadmission testing; peer review to harness doctors who habitually overtested, overdrugged, and overhospitalized their patients; and development of model treatment limits for various medical conditions. But everything was voluntary; top management was not tuned in to health care cost containment, and union leaders, who liked their jobs, were reluctant to suggest anything their members might consider a benefit reduction.

On the verge of collapse in 1979, Chrysler gingerly took its first cost-containment steps. At the company's insistence, the union

2nd opinion program

agreed to test a mandatory second-opinion program. At Chrysler's Newark, Delaware, plant, a worker whose physician recommended elective surgery was required to get from an independent physician a second opinion, which Chrysler paid for. This program reduced surgery among Newark, Delaware, employees by almost 15 percent. In 1983 Chrysler extended the program to most employees. Even though the company pays for the second opinion, the program saves Chrysler more than $1 million a year, just in health care costs.

The abuse that Chrysler most effectively addressed in the 1979 union contract concerned foot surgery. In 1978 Chrysler had paid $3.5 million to Michigan podiatrists for work on the toes, toenails, and feet of Chrysler employees and retirees and their dependents. Chrysler's medical bills for podiatry had jumped 133 percent in five years—to say nothing of the staggering disability benefits and productivity costs of absences from the job. Employees in Michigan were using foot doctors at ten times the rate of those in Illinois, nine times the rate of Alabama workers, six times the rate of those in Delaware, and four times the rate of those in Indiana. During the first quarter of 1979, Michigan podiatrists performed 16 percent of all surgery in the entire state, even though they constituted only four percent of the state's surgeons.

Chrysler's investigation revealed that some podiatrists were working on feet one toe at a visit, performing numerous unnecessary procedures, and prolonging time off the job for employees who pocketed disability benefits, which Chrysler paid at a rate of 60 percent of pay. In one case, an employee who a podiatrist claimed was disabled because of foot surgery was apprehended—after a lengthy foot chase—while attempting to steal heavy parts from a Chrysler plant. This employee had been receiving disability benefits (of $170 per week) for three weeks at the time of his arrest, and the podiatrist had reported that the employee required three more weeks off to recover.

The 1979 agreement required that Blue Cross/Blue Shield of Michigan, Chrysler's insurer, predetermine the medical necessity for foot surgery procedures suspected of most abuse. The result: a 60 percent reduction in such foot surgery and savings of more than $1 million a year in health care bills alone.

The reaction to this foot surgery program reveals a good deal about the health care business. Chrysler received not a single complaint from its workers, and none from the union. But the podiatrists sued—twice attempting to enjoin the program. Their efforts failed.

With the need and potential for health care cost savings so great and with the objective of providing health care of the same or better quality, Chrysler set up a joint committee with the UAW to work on costs. And Chrysler took a step unprecedented in American business: it created a special committee of its board of directors to tackle the health cost issue, the committee that Lee Iacocca asked me to chair.

At our initial meeting, we looked at our leverage as a large purchaser of health services. We decided to begin to reclaim the right of all consumers—and our own right, as a purchaser of health care—not to deal with unnecessarily high-priced, inefficient sellers, but to buy only from efficient ones and only the health care our employees needed.

We rejected the myth that aggressive cost controls would reduce the quality of care. Unnecessary hospitalization is an increased risk. Unnecessary surgery is an inexcusable risk. So are unnecessary X-rays, blood tests or transfusions, biopsies, and other lab tests. One of the first conclusions we reached was that cost controls and efficient health care delivery were essential to assuring our employees care of the highest quality.

We soon realized that Chrysler was then paying more than $300 million a year for health care and didn't know what it was buying or from whom. Chrysler had no idea who the efficient suppliers were, no quality controls, and no sense of how much care was truly needed by our employees.

Like most businesses, Chrysler had historically relied on whatever information its insurance carriers provided—or did not provide. Chrysler didn't know how much it was paying, for what medical tests, diagnoses, or procedures, to what doctors, hospitals, or laboratories. It had no measure of the similarities or differences among doctors or hospitals.

The first step in managing costs is to find out what they are. So we formed a health care audit staff to gather and analyze reliable information. We asked our insurance carrier for detailed information so that we could identify and then confront hospitals and doctors with unusual, unwarranted, and wasteful utilization patterns.

It wasn't easy to get Blue Cross/Blue Shield to act. But faced with our persistence, the Blues retained Health Data Institute of Newton, Massachusetts, to make a meticulous analysis of thirty months of Chrysler health care experience. Over 67,000 separate hospital admissions and more than $217 million in charges were examined. We created a computer catalogue of each incident of outpatient and inpatient care for each Chrysler employee, retiree, and dependent, by doctor and hospital. This catalogue (and a broader assessment of an even longer period) revealed a level of unnecessary care, inefficient practices, overutilization, fraud, and abuse that appalled Lee Iacocca and all Chrysler management. It provided solid evidence of wasteful spending of health benefit dollars and of diminished quality of care provided to people Chrysler insured.

From the work of the Blues and of our own audit staff, we discovered that in 1981:

- Chrysler-insured patients got more than a million laboratory tests, more than five for every insured man, woman, and child, at a cost of $12 million. (Since he hadn't had any, Iacocca quipped that "someone got at least ten.")
- Chiropractors increased over the prior year their diagnostic X-rays almost 15 percent for each employee. The Michigan Blues were billed an average of $10,000 annually per chiropractor, just for X-rays.
- In the Detroit area, the average daily cost at six of the largest acute care hospitals Chrysler employees used varied from $452 to $608. The cost for the average length of stay at these hospitals ranged from $3,028 up to $6,077—a 100 percent spread.
- The disparities were just as wide in fees different physicians charged for the same services and the tests and X-rays they prescribed for the same diagnoses.
- The single most costly medical procedure Chrysler paid for turned out to be the postadmission hospital visits—mostly that

brief bedside visit a doctor makes on his rounds—for which doctors billed Chrysler $4 million.

Hospital admissions for lower-back pain were going up at an alarming rate. We asked our physician experts to investigate eight Detroit-area hospitals with extraordinarily high percentages of nonsurgical admissions for low back problems. They found that two-thirds of the hospitalizations—and 2,264 out of 2,677 of the total hospital days (approximately 85 percent)—should never have taken place. With respect to three of the hospitals audited, not one of the admissions was found to be appropriate. The admissions, which cost Chrysler more than $1 million, turned out to be largely for "bed rest," which a patient can get more safely and inexpensively at home.

In more than 60 percent of the low back pain cases analyzed, patients were subjected to an electromyogram, an uncomfortable and expensive procedure rarely necessary for appropriate management of low back pain. Not surprisingly, every single test result was normal.

If we had any doubt about the structural defects in this fee-for-service, cost-unconscious system, our analysis of the outpatient psychiatric benefit program removed it. In 1972, Chrysler employees and retirees, and their dependents, received some 35,000 services under this program at a cost of $800,000. About that time, the proprietary psychiatric clinics in Michigan discovered the wide-open plan that Chrysler had agreed to. New ones started springing up everywhere, to solicit and serve this army of customers with the little blue-and-white card good for "free" care. By 1978 services for Chrysler-insured patients climbed to over 160,000, at a cost of $5 million. This stunning increase was arrested only when Blue Cross/Blue Shield slapped a moratorium on approving new clinics for reimbursement.

When this was reported to our health care committee, I said, "Either a disproportionate number of mentally disturbed workers are on the Chrysler payroll, or these services have given Chrysler the most mentally tranquil work force in the nation, or the psychiatrists moved to southeastern Michigan the way prospectors went West for the Gold Rush. *Or, we've got to change the system.*" What we were seeing was a perfect example of all the flawed parts of the benefit system rolled into one: (a) a hard-to-define benefit, (b) offered at no cost to employees, (c) with unlimited freedom to choose among a burgeoning network of providers attracted to money as bees are to honey, (d) who in turn had no one reviewing the need for or cost of their services. Chrysler's experience with wide-open psychiatric coverage is not unique. In 1984, after an explosion of claims for outpatient psychiatric coverage at the University of Wisconsin in Madison, Credit Life Insurance Company refused to renew the policy for students there.

Another notable example of how the "free lunch" ambience of the Chrysler plan affected patient behavior was in maternity care. Our physician-experts investigated the six Detroit-area hospitals with the highest number of maternity admissions for women insured by Chrysler. In more than 80 percent of the 618 cases studied, one or more of the hospital days were found to be unnecessary—more than 1,000 inappropriate days in all, a quarter of the total time spent in the hospital. A comparison with lengths of maternity stays in other parts of the country showed a wide divergence. The average length of stay for normal deliveries at many southern California hospitals was less than 2 days, while the Chrysler average was 3.8 days. Why shouldn't Chrysler-insured mothers choose to have an extra day or two of pampered rest when the doctor approves and it doesn't cost anything?

We discovered how charges become skewed to what the traffic will bear in such a supplier-controlled system. Among Chrysler's older retirees, and the nation's elderly in general, cataract surgery is common. This procedure takes about twenty minutes and rarely requires a general anesthetic. The average ophthalmologist charge for the operation in the Detroit area is $2,000. If a doctor performs three of these procedures a day, four days a week, forty-two weeks a year, he earns more than $1 million for less than two hundred hours of actual surgery, and has a ten-week vacation to boot. In the same metropolitan area, the average charge for serious abdominal surgery is only $1,500; such surgery takes an average of two and one-half hours—seven times as long as a typical cataract procedure—and is far riskier.

The use of dermatologists provides another example of how values become distorted in a noncompetitive supplier-controlled environment. In 1981 Blue Cross/Blue Shield payments per dermatologist were more than double those for the average practitioner, and 25 percent greater than the average payment for chest surgeons. Head for head, dermatologists grabbed more of the Michigan Blues' health insurance dollar than any other specialists did.

We also discovered that such a wide-open system is an invitation to fraud and rip-off. Chrysler worked with the FBI in an investigation of practitioners suspected of improperly certifying worker absences. In July 1981, a Detroit-area chiropractor was sent to jail for five years and fined $15,000 after pleading guilty to fifteen counts of mail fraud. He confessed to selling fake injury reports over an eighteen-month period to 1,895 auto workers, who collected $1.5 million in disability insurance payments from the Big Three automakers. He'd billed the Blues $250,000 for phony treatments and X-rays, and ordered unnecessary lab tests that cost an additional $1 million. He solicited auto workers to sell them fraudulent medical excuses; he taught them how to act during exams by insurance doctors. He charged patients $20 for work-excuse slips; $20 for each week on bogus disability, and $10 for preparing disability insurance claim forms. Those who referred other workers got an ID card entitling them to discounted prices. Often he put uninjured auto workers in body casts for a $50 charge.

Prescription drugs were also overused and abused. In a twelve-month period, a Chrysler employee obtained 51 prescriptions for 6,030 ten-milligram Valium pills. Another had 88 prescriptions filled for 4,255 five-milligram Percodans. A third obtained 136 prescriptions for four-milligram Dilaudids, totaling 8,671 tablets. That's 27 a day. All of these drugs have high street value for sale to addicts.

The need to clean up the mess was clear. If we didn't act, Chrysler's health care costs could exceed $1 billion in ten years, or $16,000 per active worker. But if Chrysler could hold projected health care costs to a growth rate even 50 percent greater than the consumer price index, it could save more than $25 million a year. Reducing the rate of increase in its health care costs just 1 percent could save the company almost $500 million over the next ten years.

With stakes so high, we've been trying hard.

One of our early efforts focused on prescription drugs. Costs for such drugs, particularly for retirees, were increasing at an alarming rate. By 1981 Chrysler's costs were $24.4 million, 8.2 percent of its total medical benefit payments. We knew we could save money by dispensing generic as opposed to brand name drugs. But Chrysler's prescription drug benefit program was not structured to encourage generic dispensing. Employees and retirees could get any prescription drug, no matter how expensive, for a $3 copayment. Chrysler paid the pharmacist for the rest of the cost of the drug dispensed, whether it was a $20 brand name product or a $7 generic equivalent.

After some hard bargaining, the United Automobile Workers agreed that Chrysler's payment to the pharmacist be limited to the price of the generic substitute, unless the providing physician prohibited substitution. If the employee wanted the brand name equivalent, he would have to pay the higher price.

In May of 1982 we launched our pilot program in Michigan with a relatively small number of drugs. Pharmacists cooperated and employee reaction was good. In the first year, Chrysler saved $250,000. We've expanded the program, and due to its success, Blue Cross/Blue Shield of Michigan has adopted the concept for all its customers. As a result, millions of dollars will be saved and the patient will get the very same health care.

Within the limits of its union contract, Chrysler has also begun to encourage outpatient surgery to save $2 million a year. The company also offered financial incentives to encourage our employees to join health maintenance organizations, which provide all the care a member needs for a price negotiated in advance.

To encourage patients to review their medical bills for accuracy, Chrysler initiated a pilot incentive program, called One Check Leads to Another. When employees or retirees find overcharges, Chrysler shares the refund with them. This program will also lead to a greater awareness on the part of our employees of the costs of their health care services, a key objective.

In January 1984 we went to the union with our findings on excess and unnecessary hospitalization, which had been confirmed by physician experts at both Health Data Institute and Blue Cross/Blue Shield of Michigan. The UAW accepted the findings. With strong union backing, we contacted offending hospitals and pressed for remedial action. Initially the atmosphere was testy, but eventually the hospitals agreed with our conclusions and committed to act and to have the progress monitored. In the six months immediately following our direct intervention at the eight hospitals with excessive admissions for lower back pain, there was a 64 percent reduction in such admissions. In the six months right after we confronted the six hospitals with the highest number of maternity cases, there was a 66 percent reduction in lengths of stay over three days for normal deliveries. For the six hospitals with routine cesarean delivery stays of seven days or more, there was a 67 percent reduction in lengths of stay over six days in the first six months after we contacted them. This analysis and intervention program proved so successful that Blue Cross/Blue Shield of Michigan has marketed it to others.

A key to lasting success is giving Chrysler-insured workers economic incentives to seek efficient health care providers. Employees respond to such incentives.

For example, under the regular Chrysler dental plan, employees must make copayments, and there is a limit beyond which the employee pays all the bills. In 1983 Chrysler introduced benefit plans in Michigan that offered employees and retirees full coverage of all dental services through dental health maintenance organizations. These plans paid the bills, with no deductibles, no copayments, and no yearly maximums. These dental groups operate like medical health maintenance organizations. They agree to perform all dental services at a fixed, prenegotiated cost to Chrysler. Since the dentists weren't operating on a fee-for-service basis, they had economic incentives to operate efficiently.

Some 11,000 Chrysler employees and retirees joined these and similar dental plans in Michigan and Indiana at the first opportunity; another 6,000 joined ten months later. They saved themselves the copayments they would have paid under the regular Chrysler-UAW dental plans and avoided the risk of having to pay amounts in excess of plan limits. They saved Chrysler close to $3 million in the first year.

Here clearly the buyers—our retirees and employees—became price-conscious and made their own choice between two types of providers. Competition and common sense worked to restructure the health care system.

The Chrysler program had a significant impact on dentists. Those who billed on a fee-for-service basis, represented by the Michigan Dental Association, mounted an organized letter-writing campaign to the homes of Chrysler employees. Dentists urged their patients not to desert the traditional system, and implied that the new system would offer care of less than top quality. In the spring of 1984, when General Motors followed Chrysler and offered a similar alternative to its employees, the community's dental association mounted a public relations campaign—with newspaper and radio advertising so distorted that a lawsuit to block it resulted in withdrawal of the ads. The *Journal of the American Dental Association* devoted its entire editorial page in July 1984 to a rebuke of me for promoting this program. Clearly, the fee-for-service dentists sense the scope of the change occurring in their business. They certainly weren't comforted by an August 13, 1984, *Forbes* magazine analysis entitled "What's Good for America Isn't Necessarily Good for the Dentists":

> When the pain of transition [to alternative systems] subsides, dentistry will probably become much like engineering. Many practitioners will work on salary. Dentists won't sink to the poverty level, but neither will they be economic aristocrats. Are the physicians listening?

Chrysler is pushing an education program for its employees and retirees on two fronts that will pay dividends in the long run. First, we've mounted a major health-promotion and disease-prevention effort to keep people out of the hospital and in good health. We inform our people about the dangers of smoking and urge them to quit. We tell them about the benefits of proper diet, exercise, and

rest, and the dangers of alcohol abuse. We provide financial incentives to adopt healthy life-styles. More than one executive quit
smoking upon learning that company life insurance rates were 75
percent higher for smokers. Second, we tell our workers—and top
executives—about the waste and inefficiency in the health care
system and, most important, about the fact that they can make
choices and get better or equally fine health care at far less cost.
We do this through special presentations, our company publications, and a regular newspaper feature we've created for this purpose called *Health Talk.*

But Chrysler has achieved immediate savings with a program in
Michigan to screen hospital admissions and control lengths of stay
for Chrysler's nonunion employees. All nonemergency, nonmaternity cases require a second, independent medical opinion before
admission, and each is limited to a specific length of stay in the absence of unforeseen complications. If the admitting physician believes the stay should be extended beyond the specified period, he
must go to Blue Cross in advance, explain why, and get approval.
Otherwise, Blue Cross will not pay for the extra time. The savings
hit $2 million in the first year.

Chrysler's health care cost-containment effort has had real success. In 1982 and prior years, actual costs invariably exceeded
budget estimates. Costs in 1983 were $20 million under Chrysler's
original budget, owing largely to reduced hospitalization. In 1983
the company's forecast of health care expenditures for 1984 was
$460 million. But throughout the year we reduced utilization of
both hospital and physician services. These reductions were the
results of several action plans: Chrysler's own efforts, the actions
of other businesses, the fallout from Medicare's bold stroke in establishing diagnosis related groups (a plan that sets hospital payments in advance for 470 separate diagnoses), a general awakening
of Chrysler employees and retirees about the issues, and a positive
reaction from providers.

By the end of 1984, Chrysler had spent $402 million for health
care—a $58 million reduction below our budget!

Reducing hospitalization, more than any other single effort, was
responsible for the enormous savings in 1984. Of the $58 million
saved, we believe that about $32 million is attributable to hospital

costs, and about $22 million to doctors' fees and tests largely associated with hospitalization. The remaining $4 million comes from the acceptance of dental HMOs, our move to generic drugs, and other cost-cutting activities.

The most important lesson from the Chrysler experience is not that $58 million was saved in 1984. The gospel lesson is that hard-negotiating buyers, who treat health care like the other products they purchase, can change the system—and we are only beginning to realize the benefits of competition.

Where this comes through most clearly in the Chrysler experience is in what's happened to Blue Cross/Blue Shield premiums compared with the price of health maintenance organizations. For Chrysler's salaried employees, we have been able to put in place all changes as soon as they appeared to make sense. As a result, for salaried employees, in 1985 the Michigan Blue Cross/Blue Shield premiums were lower than the charges of Detroit health maintenance organizations. Because we have not been able to make all the changes for our union employees, Blue Cross/Blue Shield premiums for them were still higher than HMO charges—but we have been closing the gap. The largest single reason is that we are wringing unnecessary hospitalization out of the Blue Cross/Blue Shield plan. We have already approached Michigan HMOs and asked them to reduce their charges to us.

In 1985 we began preparing an effort to confront physicians, as we have hospitals, to ask those who charge twice as much or more for the same services why they do so, to redress the imbalance of skewed payments for cataract operations and dermatology as opposed to charges for general surgery and the services of family physicians, to establish professional screens, cost-benefit standards and specific lengths of treatment for psychiatric care, to seek out the most efficient hospitals, doctors, dentists, laboratories, and radiologists and give our business to them.

Ironically, some of the greatest resistance to changing the health care system has come from the United Automobile Workers leadership. The union, which publicly espouses massive restructuring of our system into a national health plan that would sharply curtail freedom of choice, has sought to perpetuate the freedom-of-choice myth in its private negotiations. Sitting across from me when I was Secretary of HEW, Douglas Fraser, then president of the UAW, used to put down my concern about the political reaction of Congress to any national health plan that restricted individual freedom to select any doctor or hospital. "We'll all have to learn that you can't have complete freedom of choice. You can't have everything . . . and access to care for all is the important thing," he told me on more than one occasion.

Sitting across the union bargaining table, with Chrysler management arguing that workers who choose more expensive, less efficient doctors and health care providers should pay the extra cost and those who join less expensive prepaid plans should get some of the savings, UAW negotiators cry foul. They have argued: you can't take unlimited freedom of choice away from our members; making them pay more for fee-for-service doctors does that; the workers won't stand for it. In business and labor, as in government bureaucracy, where one stands depends on where one sits.

Chrysler and the other auto companies have tried to convince the UAW that competitive delivery systems can give their members the same full range of benefits they have today. Chrysler and other employers can negotiate agreements with efficient doctors, hospitals, and other health care providers, either directly or through a number of organizations, to deliver quality health services at prearranged lower prices.

Chrysler studies clearly indicated that the premiums for coverage delivered by such an efficient network would be far less than those for coverage under typical first-dollar, open-access plans. To make the system work most effectively, the employer's contributions for any such plan should be limited to the cost of the most efficient plan; employees choosing a more expensive plan should pay the added cost, through either an additional premium or some form of cost sharing. This would inject price competition into the consumer health care equation, get employees to consider cost when making their health plan decisions, and assure efficient providers that employees would have a real incentive to join the new plan.

Union leaders have been reluctant to encourage their members to agree to a new system. They have argued that, while large numbers of doctors and hospitals might participate in alternative delivery systems, not all would. Some might choose not to. Those who were inefficient or costly would not be permitted to. So some workers might have to change doctors or pay additional costs, and union leaders contend that this would inhibit their members' "freedom of choice." These arguments from the union could come as easily from the lips of the American Medical Association. But members who wanted more expensive doctors could have them if they paid the extra cost—just as now they can have a private hospital room if they pay the extra cost.

Chrysler unsuccessfully proposed this kind of alternative to the UAW during its 1982 negotiations. The aura of "no more concessions" that clouded those talks guaranteed rejection. But there may be hope, since UAW leaders have taken steps toward fostering competition in the delivery of health care in the 1984 aerospace-industry and the 1984 and 1985 auto-industry contracts.

In its 1984 contract with Rockwell International, the UAW bargaining team helped develop a new program similar to Chrysler's 1982 proposal. The Rockwell plan offers employees three health care options: health maintenance organizations, preferred provider organizations, or a "90/10" plan.

The first two options provide comprehensive health care services at little or no charge to the patient. The "90/10" plan is a fee-for-service, open access plan: the worker pays an up-front deductible and 10 percent of each bill thereafter for choosing this, the most expensive plan. All plans mandate a review of all care in hospitals to assure quality and cost-effective treatment there.

The 1984 UAW/Rockwell contract contains other key features. All new employees must join HMOs for at least the first year. To limit increases in Rockwell's expenses for retiree coverage as a result of Medicare cost shifting, Rockwell's liability is frozen at July 1, 1984, levels. If, after that date, Medicare increases cost sharing for its beneficiaries or reduces their benefits, Rockwell does not pick up the tab unless it so agrees in new negotiations.

Unfortunately, the 1984 contracts between the UAW and General Motors and Ford did not go nearly so far as the Rockwell contracts in promoting the development of competitive alternative delivery systems. Those agreements did provide alternative care systems for workers, but because they continued to offer first-dollar, fee-for-service, unlimited-choice coverage at no extra cost, workers had no incentive to select a more efficient system. At General Motors, only 16 percent of the employees and retirees chose a more efficiently managed care system; the rest continued in the traditional fee-for-service plan. The GM and Ford contracts do include cost-containment measures for that plan, the most important of which is a requirement for preauthorization by the insurer before providing full coverage of nonmaternity or nonemergency hospitalization. If such hospitalization is not approved in advance, the patient pays a deductible and a portion of the bill above the deductible.

In the three-year contract signed in October 1985, Chrysler and the United Automobile Workers agreed to a wide range of cost containment measures that saved at least $50 million while providing employees even higher-quality health care.

- Beginning in early 1986, union members became subject to the same hospital prescreening program as other Chrysler employees. The need for admission is now certified and a maximum length of stay determined in advance. If prior approval is not obtained for admission or for extending a stay, Blue Cross will not pay. This step alone saves about $10 million a year.

- Employees were offered a preferred provider health plan, to compete with the current Blue Cross/Blue Shield and HMO options.

- Starting in Michigan, Chrysler fully paid for certain health care benefits previously covered under the Blue Cross/Blue Shield plan only if delivered through specialists that Chrysler contracts with. These benefits include vision care and podiatry services. Employees and their doctors have a powerful financial incentive to use these preferred providers; going to others requires employees to make substantial copayments.

- Chrysler solicited bids from laboratories that wanted to perform outpatient tests on its employees. The lowest bidder became the only lab Chrysler will pay. Doctors who don't use that lab have to pay for the tests themselves or charge their Chrysler patients.

- Dental HMOs, already available to employees in Michigan, Illinois, and Indiana, were extended to workers in Ohio, Missouri, Delaware, New York, and Alabama.

- A joint Chrysler-UAW committee set up other specialized preferred providers—for psychiatric services, substance abuse, and prescription drugs.

- The Chrysler-UAW group will seek ways to avoid unnecessary emergency-room use.

In another 1985 development that gives a sense of what the future may hold for health care in America, the UAW accepted managed care only—through health maintenance organizations or preferred providers—for its workers at the new General Motors Saturn and NUMMI plants.

Despite Chrysler's efforts, its 1984 health care costs still topped $400 million—that's more than $1 million each day—and the Blues remained Chrysler's largest single supplier. When we include Chrysler's $22 million share of the Medicare payroll tax and a portion of the health insurance premiums of its suppliers, Chrysler's total 1984 health care bill exceeded $530 for each car sold. That's almost 10 percent of the cost of the lowest-priced models. It's seven times the $75 a car that health care cost Chrysler in 1970. The number is down somewhat from $600 a car in 1983—not so much because the inflation in health care costs abated in 1984 as because we cut hospitalization and we're selling more cars. In 1984 Chrysler had to sell about 70,000 vehicles just to pay its health care bills.

What does Chrysler's health care bill mean to its workers?

In 1984 the average hourly worker had to produce more than $5,000 in revenues just to pay for health care. That amount equals what he was paid for almost three months of work. In 1972 the comparable amount—$850—was equal to less than one month's pay. Chrysler's 1984 health care bill exceeded the amount Chrysler paid in cash retirement benefits to all 65,000 of its pensioners and was four times what it paid its stockholders in dividends.

Chrysler's health care costs erode its ability to compete with Japanese and other foreign car makers. Mitsubishi Motor Corporation, a Japanese car manufacturer in which Chrysler has an investment, spent only $880 for an employee's health care cost in 1984, while each employee paid approximately $408. Chrysler's comparable cost per active employee is more than 400 percent higher. Unlike Chrysler, Mitsubishi had no direct cost for retirees or their surviving spouses because of Japan's national health coverage.

There's plenty more to do at Chrysler, but its dramatic savings underscore the importance of having a variety of delivery systems compete for the dollar of an aroused business community.

I have recounted the Chrysler story here because I've lived it. The experience has led me to develop enormous respect for the genius of American business and a competitive private sector. I have watched businesses grapple with this problem with imagination and determination and freedom to act, not inhibited, as government often is, by politics and the power of special interest groups. Indeed, business is key to solving the health care cost crisis in America.

Its stake is enormous. American businesses spent about $90 billion in health insurance premiums in 1984, 38 percent of their 1984 pretax profits, more than they paid in dividends to their shareholders.

The Big Three auto companies alone spent $3.5 billion for health care in 1984. That's more than each of thirty-two states collected in taxes and spent that year.

Business has the drive and motivation to tackle this problem. In the American tradition, it has already deployed hundreds of independent minds and skills, all across our nation, to experiment and seek solutions.

American business abounds with revolutionaries who are already changing our health care delivery system. R. J. Reynolds Industries has established its own health maintenance medical and dental organizations, with their own pharmacy, in Winston-Salem,

North Carolina. They serve 87 percent of the Reynolds-covered population and have provided top-quality health care, with a 50 percent reduction in hospitalization and a 90 percent reduction in emergency-room use. The dental facility's emphasis on preventive care has allowed Reynolds to reduce the number of dentists needed to serve its people. Commercial insurers and the Blues estimate that a fully insured fee-for-service program with comparable medical and dental benefits would cost 40 to 45 percent more. The glut of dentists makes plans like this feasible for many corporations. Reynolds has held its annual rate of increase in health care costs to 6 or 7 percent, while regular insurance plans have been averaging 15 to 20 percent premium hikes each year. (Just think of what Reynolds could achieve if it mounted a campaign to get its employees to quit smoking!)

In 1984 Pillsbury Company began negotiating fees with doctors and hospitals before treatment, "to make sure our employees get the kind of rates they ought to get."

Quaker Oats cut its medical premium year-to-year increase from 20 percent in 1982 to 4 percent in 1983 by shifting from first-dollar, "free lunch" coverage for which employees paid nothing to a plan under which they paid 15 percent of health care bills. PepsiCo attributes its less than 10 percent increases in health insurance costs year to year to its insistence that through deductibles, copayments, and premium sharing, workers pay 40 percent of the company's health care costs. Some 63 percent of corporations of all sizes in one survey moved to some cost sharing to make their employees conscious of the cost of health care in 1984; only 30 percent had any cost sharing in 1982.

Berol Corporation in Danbury, Connecticut, requires employees to get a second opinion for fourteen specific operations or else pay half the cost of the surgery themselves. It offers employees who have filed no health claims $500 per year; those who file claims totaling under $500 get the difference. Since putting this plan into effect in 1983, Berol has experienced no increase in health insurance premiums and expects none through 1986.

When doctors and hospitals in Lawton, Oklahoma, refused to negotiate fees and charges with Goodyear Tire & Rubber, the company built a $180,000 medical clinic at its plant, with doctors, laboratory, and pharmacy. The prices are half what medical offices in Lawton charge.

Business is also becoming conscious of the competitive disadvantages of higher health care costs. Take defense contractors: in 1984 Boeing Company in Seattle paid for hospital rooms at half the rate that McDonnell-Douglas Corporation paid in St. Louis.

Hewlett-Packard is testing a total-package, "global" payment system, in which the company pays a single amount for everything required to perform gall bladder and hernia operations—hospital bills, physicians' fees, nurses, laboratory tests.

Owens-Illinois, Incorporated, faced with annual hikes of 18 percent in health insurance premiums, redesigned its plan to increase employee deductibles and premium payments, discourage the use of expensive hospital care where outpatient services would do just as well (for example, by reversing a plan that had paid full cost for tests done in the hospital and only partial costs for those done outside the hospital), and require a second opinion before the company would pay the full bill for certain surgery. The cost of the second-opinion program in its first year was $137,000. But the net savings to Owens-Illinois was more than $400,000. The company has also instituted a Well Worth It program to encourage employees to eat properly, quit smoking, and get proper exercise. The result of all of this: the company actually reduced total health care costs from $120 million in 1982 to $114 million in 1983, an impressive reversal of the 46 percent increase over the preceding five years.

Several companies now require doctors to submit treatment plans that include hospitalization in advance to independent professionals, who determine, under company guidelines, whether the illness is covered for hospitalization and, if so, how many days will be paid for.

Caterpillar Tractor Company started a hospital utilization review program that cut hospital admissions by 10 percent, hospital stays by 12 percent, and total days of hospital care by 18.4 percent. At Public Service Electric & Gas Company of New Jersey, preadmission testing reduced hospital stays for surgical admissions by an average of 3.8 days, and for medical admissions by an average of 2.3 days.

John Deere and Company's program to require preauthorization for inpatient oral surgery and to offer pricing incentives for outpatient surgery has slashed admissions for that procedure by 75 percent.

The percentage of blue-chip Business Roundtable companies offering employees financial incentives to have outpatient rather than inpatient surgery has jumped from 4 to 40 from 1982 to 1984. Most large employers have made significant changes in their health care plans since 1982; 54 percent added coverage of second opinions before surgery, more than half added or increased deductibles, 47 percent adopted measures to stem unnecessary hospitalization, and 34 percent added some managed-care option to fee-for-service plans, such as a health maintenance organization.

Perhaps the most revolutionary approach to cost containment is keeping workers healthy, rather than simply paying for their care after they're sick. Since 1979, Johnson and Johnson has been mounting the most ambitious employee health-promotion and disease-prevention effort in America. The payoff has been big for the company and its workers. By 1985, Johnson and Johnson's Live for Life program involved 30,000 employees at fifty locations in the United States, Puerto Rico, and Europe. More than 90 percent of these employees got an initial health screening. Sixty percent participated in one or more of the program's six core elements: smoking cessation, weight control, nutrition, exercise, blood pressure control, and stress management. All employees, even those not in the program, are repeatedly urged to adopt healthy life-styles.

Johnson and Johnson reports these early results:

- 25 percent of all employees who smoked in 1980 had stopped by 1982; 40 percent of the smokers in the program had stopped.
- The average heart efficiency of all employees increased 11 percent over a two-year period—more than halfway toward the 20 percent maximum increase any individual can achieve.
- The average blood pressure of all employees dropped by three points.
- Hospital costs plummeted 35 percent.
- Absenteeism went down 15 to 20 percent.

The cost at different work sites varied from $150 to $200 a year for each employee. By the third year of operation at a work site the program broke even, with spending offset by savings from reduced absenteeism and lower health care costs. By the fifth year, the company's total investment was paid off, and in the sixth, savings per employee reached three times costs. Moreover, Johnson and Johnson has found that its program boosts employee morale and job satisfaction.

Central to the Live for Life effort is saturation marketing, and a recognition that exercise and other health-promoting activities compete for an employee's time and loyalty against alternatives like a longer lunch with a couple of beers and a few minutes more sleep in the morning. With this in mind, Johnson and Johnson has used the same marketing expertise it uses to sell baby powder and cotton swabs.

The Chrysler story and the awakening of many other corporations like Johnson and Johnson indicate that we can do something about our health care cost crisis. But business alone cannot control health care costs. There is work for each of us in restructuring our health care system. The first task is to understand how we planted the seeds that threaten the best of our health care system and the civility of our society.

Chapter 3

HOW DID WE GET HERE?

Can we have the miracles of modern medicine without the colossal costs, inefficiency, waste, and abuse?

Of course.

Well, then, how did we get into this mess?

We all contributed mightily, and most of the time we acted with the best of intentions, without foreseeing the worst of the unintended effects.

Our actions have been taken in the wake of our nation's public health triumphs in the early twentieth century. The major health care struggle in America as the nineteenth century gave way to the twentieth was against infectious diseases.

At the beginning of the twentieth century, the leading causes of death in the United States were tuberculosis, diphtheria, influenza, pneumonia, cholera, and gastrointestinal infections. In 1900 there were 580 deaths from these major infectious diseases for every 100,000 Americans. Over the next few decades, we mounted major public health strategies against these diseases: sewer and sanitation systems, pasteurization of milk, effective vaccines, and mass immunization programs. These advances were foremost in driving down the infant mortality rate from 140 for each 1,000 babies born in 1900 to 65 for each 1,000 born in 1930.

The mid-1930s saw the introduction of the "wonder drugs": first the sulfa drugs and then penicillin, streptomycin, and a host of others. From 1935 to 1950 infant mortality dropped at an annual rate of 4.3 percent; the overall death rate from influenza and pneumonia dropped twice as fast.

As a result, in 1984 these infectious diseases accounted for less than 30 deaths for every 100,000 Americans. Indeed, in the mid-1980s the major killers of the first part of this century are hard to find. Infant mortality is down to 10.6 deaths for each 1,000 babies born. We have eliminated smallpox through the world. We are within close reach of eliminating measles as an indigenous disease in the United States, and we can eventually do the same global job on measles and other childhood diseases that we've done on smallpox.

As death from the acute infectious diseases plummeted, new killers and maimers, among them heart disease, cancer, and stroke, increased their toll on human life. By 1984 cardiovascular ailments, notably including heart disease and stroke, were responsible for half the deaths in America. Cancer was second, the cause of 22 percent of American mortalities. Accidents, often precipitated by alcohol abuse, produced 5 percent of America's deaths and exacted a fearsome cost in disability. Respiratory diseases, like chronic bronchitis and emphysema, and alcoholism have also taken their places high on the death charts.

The revolution in public health and the ascendancy of new killing and crippling diseases formed the background against which the forces for health care cost increases gathered. If sanitary engineering, scientific invention, and miracle vaccines vastly reduced infectious diseases, they also generated revolutionary changes in our perceptions—and the reality—of hospitals and doctors.

Until the twentieth century, hospitals were places where people died. An 1870 English study concluded that the death rate from surgery was higher in the hospital than in the home. Doctors could ease pain with morphine and sometimes reduce symptoms, but they had no miracle drugs to prescribe. Indeed, individuals could buy virtually any drug without a prescription, so the doctor wasn't even needed to write one. More often than not, the physician's main role was to console the afflicted and the family and help find the priest to give the last rites.

Beginning in the last quarter of the nineteenth century and accelerating as the twentieth century moved along, a change occurred in these perceptions and realities. Antiseptics were discovered, aseptic practices introduced. Hospitals greatly improved their sanitary conditions, and after surgical operations more people came home and fewer went to the graveyard. As survival rates rose, the practice of surgery mushroomed. The famous Mayo brothers, who did only 54 abdominal operations in the four years from 1889 through 1892, performed more than 2,000 in 1905. As hospitals became the workplaces for surgeons, their number increased from 178 in 1872 to 4,000 in 1910, to nearly 7,000 in 1980. In 1821 only three hospitals were expressly devoted to curing illnesses; the rest were basically dormitories for the sick. Today virtually all hospitals engage in therapeutic pursuits. Hospitals got more expensive as they shifted from giving the indigent long-term custodial care in large wards to providing paying surgical patients medical services in semiprivate and private rooms. Hospital construction costs rose from less than $1,000 per bed in 1870 to $150,000 in 1984.

A no less dramatic shift occurred in our view of doctors, and their sense of themselves. We began to look upon them as healers rather than pain relievers, and they began to look after their newfound economic and social status. And they moved to get field position.

Doctors organized state medical societies, and forged the American Medical Association into an effective national political instrument. Founded in 1845, the AMA had little influence at the turn of the century; only 8,000 of America's 100,000 doctors even bothered to join. By 1910 the AMA claimed 70,000 members, about half the doctors in America. Organized along state lines, the association created potent political action groups, alerted the public to the false claims of many patent medicines, and became a force to reckon with in the legislative and regulatory process, national and local. In 1984 the AMA had 217,000 members, 43 percent of America's doctors. /

In the self-interest of doctors and in the public interest of patients, the AMA had begun in 1905 to refuse to accept ads in its journal for any therapeutic drug that was advertised directly to the public. Sparked by the need to protect people against snake-oil drummers and quacks exposed by muckraking reporters—and with hearty encouragement from medical associations—states and the national government made the doctor's prescription the indispensable key to patient access to most drugs. Then, over the mid–twentieth century, scientists discovered and pharmaceutical companies marketed a legion of miracle drugs for everything from respiratory diseases to depression, stress, high blood pressure, and diabetes. The doctors were perfectly positioned with the keys to the miracle drug kingdom, the exclusive power to prescribe.

The AMA also supported the work of Abraham Flexner, who in 1910 exposed the false claims and shoddy curriculum, facilities, and faculties of many medical schools. The public outcry over Flexner's revelations gave decisive momentum to state enactment of stiffer licensing requirements for physicians. In the five years following the Flexner report, 62 of the 131 medical schools in the country closed down, and the number of new graduates fell 35 percent, from 5,440 to 3,536. The national supply of physicians—in 1900, one for every 578 Americans—declined to one for every 730 Americans by 1920.

Over this same period, states passed laws severely restricting to physicians trained at accredited schools the "practice of medicine," a phrase broadly defined, to protect the public from quacks and charlatans. Because it was taken for granted that doctors knew best about medicine and science, these laws often delegated sweeping regulatory power to state medical societies. Little attention was paid to the control over the marketplace that these statutes vested in physicians. But the evidence was there: while overall consumer prices doubled between 1900 and 1928, the incomes of physicians quadrupled, and doctors, whose average nineteenth-century income had put them in the lower middle class in America, began their climb up the stairway to paradise of status and money in America.

Soon, to speak the words "my son the doctor" became the prayer and dream of a generation of immigrants. After all, doctors were professionals and they took the Hippocratic oath, which, though quaint in the context of modern medicine, is worth setting forth in its pristine entirety:

> I swear by Apollo the physician, by Aesculapius, Hygeia, and Panacea, and I take to witness all the gods, all the goddesses, to keep according to my ability and my judgment the following Oath:
>
> To consider dear to me as my parents him who taught me this art; to live in common with him and if necessary to share my goods with him; to look upon his children as my own brothers, to teach them this art if they so desire without fee or written promise; to impart to my sons and the sons of the master who taught me and the disciples who have enrolled themselves and have agreed to the rules of the profession, but to these alone, the precepts and the instruction. I will prescribe regimen for the good of my patients according to my ability and my judgment and never do harm to anyone. To please no one will I prescribe a deadly drug, nor give advice which may cause his death. Nor will I give a woman a pessary to produce abortion. But I will preserve the purity of my life and my art. I will not cut for stone, even for patients in whom the disease is manifest; I will leave this operation to be performed by practitioners (specialists in this art). In every house where I come I will enter only for the good of my patients, keeping myself far from all intentional ill-doing and all seduction, and especially from the pleasures of love with women or with men, be they free or slaves. All that may come to my knowledge in the exercise of my profession or in daily commerce with men, which ought not to be spread abroad, I will keep secret and will never reveal. If I keep this oath faithfully, may I enjoy my life and practice my art, respected by all men and in all times; but if I swerve from it or violate it, may the reverse be my lot.

By the late 1920s the hard core of today's health industry—physicians, hospitals, medical education, state licensing, and some early medical research successes—was pretty much in place. What was needed was to plant a medical money tree, a system to finance the business of medicine and health care.

Prior to the 1930s there was virtually no health insurance in the United States. Americans personally paid more than 90 percent of their hospital and doctors' bills. What coverage existed aimed at replacing some part of wages lost due to illness or accident. There was little sentiment for health insurance, partly because, unlike Europe, America had no tradition of broad social insurance schemes, and partly because the need was not perceived as acute. Physicians' charges were low and hospitals still provided lots of charitable care.

From 1913 to 1919 a modest effort to promote national health insurance had some early support from the American Medical Association and the business community. But the attempt sputtered for lack of popular support, and the proposal was eventually opposed not only by business and the AMA but by Samuel Gompers, president of the American Federation of Labor. The great labor leader saw it as a threat to union-sponsored insurance programs, which helped build membership.

In the 1920s hospital costs began to rise, particularly those for extended stays. By 1929 illnesses requiring hospitalization accounted for 50 percent of all medical expenditures. Then the Great Depression struck and people went to hospitals only in dire emergencies. Many patients couldn't pay their bills. Between 1929 and 1930, average hospital receipts plummeted from more than $200 per patient to less than $60.

Spurred by the ravages of the depression, potential patients and hospital administrators began to look for some way to pay and be paid. And health insurance became an industry within the health industry.

It started in 1929 in Dallas, Texas. Baylor University Hospital initiated an insurance plan for 1,250 schoolteachers. Each teacher paid fifty cents a month and received up to twenty-one days of hospital care each year. Other Dallas hospitals soon offered competing plans, and the idea spread to cities across America.

Three years later, in 1932, a community-wide plan was developed in California. Under it, participating hospitals in a given area agreed to provide services to subscribers, who paid their premiums to the plan rather than to individual hospitals. The community-wide concept eliminated any competition among the participating hospitals; there was no need for each to provide its own plan. Hospitals in other areas embraced such plans and marketed them on a not-for-profit basis. They became known as Blue Cross plans. By 1937 these noncompetitive plans had 800,000 subscribers, while competing plans set up by individual hospitals had only 125,000. In 1938 the American Hospital Association began vigorously promoting noncompetitive community-wide Blue Cross plans; by 1940 membership ballooned to six million.

These Blue Cross plans covered only hospitalization and offered a single community rate, regardless of the risk related to specific groups and individuals. Participating hospitals guaranteed to provide the stipulated services to members of Blue Cross plans. Organized and administered by community groups and hospitals, these not-for-profit plans were exempt from taxes.

Initially, commercial insurers were wary of health insurance because of the difficulty of establishing actuarial principles that would ensure a profit. As Blue Cross plans succeeded, however, commercial insurers began to offer coverage, in 1934 for hospitalization, in 1939 for surgery. Commercial insurers did not use a single community-wide risk rate; they calculated rates based upon their experience related to differences in age and health. Typically, commercial policies offered cash payments to individual subscribers, rather than paying hospitals directly, as Blue Cross did. The cash patients received from these commercial insurance plans could be used to pay doctors as well as hospitals. By 1940 commercial insurers covered 3.7 million people.

The American Medical Association did not object to commercial insurers paying cash to patients, who in turn paid doctors. But the association initially resisted any health plans that paid physicians directly, considering such plans corrosive of the doctor-patient relationship.

Blue Cross plans, which covered only hospitalization and not doctors' bills, began to look for ways to compete with commercial insurers. At the same time, physicians were seeking ways to take the steam out of proposals in some states, like California, for mandatory government health insurance to cover doctors' and hospital bills. Working together in the late 1930s and early 1940s, Blue Cross organizations and physicians established Blue Shield plans to complement Blue Cross hospitalization with coverage of physicians' services. In the beginning, these plans offered subscribers cash payments for doctors' hospital fees only. Eventually, physicians' services of all sorts were covered and the AMA eased its objection to direct payments to doctors.

Both Blue Cross and Blue Shield were captives of the doctors and hospitals. Through their state and local medical societies and their dominance of the boards of directors of the Blues, doctors controlled the scope of coverage and the amounts they and the hospitals were paid. Portrayed as a public service, Blue Shield was also a minimum income security program for doctors. Participating doctors had to accept the amounts the plans set as full payment only for low-income subscribers; they were free to levy additional charges on others. Doctors who chose not to participate could charge Blue Shield subscribers at any income level whatever they wished for a particular service. The patients then had to make up the difference between the doctors' charge and what Blue Shield paid.

The commercial plans were initially independent of doctors and hospitals. They frequently contested the unfair advantage of Blue Cross and Blue Shield plans that physicians controlled. But at this stage, commercial insurers were not about to jeopardize their business by getting involved with what doctors or hospitals charged. Within a short time, commercial plans perceived themselves as more closely aligned with the doctors and hospitals whose bills they paid than with the patients who bought their insurance.

The patients, who were the consumers of health care, were dazzled by the magic of the medicine men and grateful for some protection. Before these consumers realized what was happening, or anybody took much notice, the health insurance sector of the health care industry was harnessed to minimize competition, control prices, direct usage, and ease bill collection for doctors and hospitals. In the case of Blue Cross and Blue Shield, the hospitals and the doctors controlled rates, coverage, and payment; in the case of commercial plans that paid patients directly, there were no limits on charges by hospitals or doctors.

Big Corporate America and Big Union America were not paying much attention to these developments either. After all, what did the employment relationship have to do with health insurance benefits in a world where child labor protection laws were barely making it through Congress and union organizing was a dirty, often violent business that threatened the lives of men like UAW president Walter Reuther?

World War II changed all that. Price and wage controls were strictly enforced and observed. As pressure mounted for pay increases, the War Labor Board held the line on wages, but it did permit increases in fringe benefits in amounts equivalent to 5 percent of wages. Health insurance became a premier fringe benefit. Employers began to use group health insurance to attract scarce labor, and unions began to regard such insurance as a way to supplement income. The tax laws provided added stimulus: unlike wages and most other fringe benefits, employer contributions to group health insurance policies were tax-deductible business expenses, were explicitly exempted from employees' taxable income, and were not subject to the payroll taxes shared by employers and employees. The number of Americans enrolled in group hospital plans bolted from seven million in 1942 to twenty-six million by the end of the war.

Corporate employers tended to prefer commercial insurers to Blue Cross and Blue Shield because the commercial insurers based their rates on the age and health of the particular group covered. For most corporations, this meant lower rates. Commercial insurers also offered more flexibility and variety in types of coverage, and they were quick to work out arrangements so that the employer could take full credit with its employees for providing the benefits. Eventually, as the corporate group insurance market expanded, Blue Cross and Blue Shield began adjusting their plans for employers in an attempt to compete with commercial insurance companies.

In 1947 Congress passed the Taft-Hartley Labor Relations Act, a legislative rule book for labor-management relations. In 1949, in the *Inland Steel* case, the United States Supreme Court ruled that certain fringe benefits, including health care plans, were among the collective bargaining issues the act gave unions the right to negotiate. And negotiate they did. The number of union workers covered by health plans went from 2.7 million, with spotty protection for dependents, before *Inland Steel* to 12 million workers and all their 17 million dependents just six years later.

As employers negotiated health care packages with unionized employees, commercial insurers surpassed Blue Cross in hospitalization coverage. Because the focus of employer-employee insurance was expensive catastrophic care, the insurance benefits first bargained for were tilted decidedly toward hospital care. As unions gained power, however, big corporations agreed to coverage for outpatient physician care, prescription drugs, and laboratory tests. In the early rounds of bargaining, corporations insisted that employees pay some part of the health insurance premiums and doctors' and hospital bills.

Then the large unions mounted a major effort to reduce payments by employees toward their health insurance premiums and health care bills.

The big event came in 1959. A 116-day United Steelworkers strike ended with a settlement that required the steel companies to pay the entire premium for health insurance. In 1961 General Motors, Ford, and Chrysler accepted similar health care schemes in their negotiations with the United Automobile Workers. The three auto companies agreed to pay the full cost of hospital, surgical, and medical insurance premiums for employees and their dependents. Throughout the 1960s and 1970s, business and labor kept extending health insurance coverage and benefits and eliminating worker incentives to seek efficient care and physician incentives to hold down fees and hospitalization.

Without appreciating the full implications, big business and big labor signaled the fall from grace of deductible plans, under which the employee paid a certain amount of doctors' or hospital bills before the insurance company took over the payments, and of copayment plans, under which the employee paid a share (usually 20 percent) of each doctor's or hospital bill. The first-dollar coverage plans, as they became known, rendered the cost of the doctor or hospital irrelevant to any patient they insured.

First-dollar coverage plans spread like an infectious flu through a crowded elementary school—not only among union employees, but among nonorganized white-collar workers as well. By and large, employers could not easily give greater benefits to union employees than to nonunion workers. Companies without unions wanted to stay that way, and one method was to provide good wages and generous fringe benefits, to convince employees that they had all the advantages of being organized, without the need to pay union dues. Moreover, as corporate and individual income and payroll taxes increased, deductible, nontaxable health care benefits became better than money. The employment relationship became the source of health care benefits for virtually all working Americans and their families.

To a great extent, the health industry was insulated from the competing demands of food, clothing, shelter, and recreation on a family budget. Its cost was hidden in the products consumers bought—from cars and radios to food, clothing, and shelter themselves. Families blanketed in the rich first-dollar coverage plans thought they never had to pay for doctors or hospitals.

Remarkably, in negotiating health care plans big companies and big unions did not agree to dollar amounts, as they did in all other aspects of their bargaining. With little apparent concern, companies promised to provide benefits, whatever the cost. After all, it seemed a lot less expensive to give employees health care than a higher per-hour wage, and unions kept demanding more health care coverage for their members. Throughout the post–World War II period, with each round of bargaining, managers who fought with other suppliers over the price of each nail or screw and union leaders who negotiated for each half-cent an hour kept adding health benefits to contracts, without realizing that they were becoming hostage to costs beyond their control—costs that over the long run would jeopardize jobs and hobble profits.

Such was the stage set for the government as it debated in the early 1960s whether to enact some kind of national health plan. About 60 percent of our citizens, 110 million Americans, were at least partially insulated from hospital and doctors' bills; many didn't have to pay much or anything. Our biggest corporations and unions had, with little or no appreciation of the ramifications, granted to doctors, hospital administrators, medical laboratories, and pharmaceutical manufacturers the power to tell the patients what services, tests, and drugs to buy, regardless of cost. The steel

and auto workers, other big unions, and the Fortune 500—the
tough streetfighters of labor and business—had been kidnapped by
the health care industry without so much as a whimper. They
didn't even know what had happened until it was too late.

The national government's role in health care was marginal up
to World War II. True, the Public Health Service was established
in 1789, as the Marine Hospital Service, to serve merchant seamen
and Navy personnel. At the turn of the century, Congress began
expanding the mission of the Public Health Service to include the
study of infectious diseases and control of epidemics. President
Franklin Delano Roosevelt briefly considered shoehorning health
care benefits into the Social Security proposals he presented to
Congress in 1935, but he dropped the idea for fear of losing the
basic retirement-income package.

As part of the nation's mobilization for World War II, the federal government was required to make substantial investments in
health care training and medical research. The armed forces
needed physicians and nurses, so they drafted all they could get
their hands on and trained even more. Medical research was conducted on everything from frostbite to malaria to venereal disease
to surgical and burn procedures.

Much of that effort, somewhat redirected, continued after the
war, and research became the first medical arena Uncle Sam en-
tered on a major scale.

The National Institute of Health, created in 1930, started with a
budget of less than $50,000. At the end of World War II, the mul-
timillion-dollar military medical research effort was transferred
there. In 1944 Congress gave the U.S. Surgeon General sweeping
powers to support research in the diseases and disabilities of man
and authorized a variety of projects and fellowships. By 1947 the
National Institutes of Health (NIH) had become the nation's major
center for medical research, with a budget of $8 million. By 1960
the medical research budget of the National Institutes of Health
had multiplied fiftyfold, to an annual total of $400 million; by
1984 it topped $4 billion.

Much of NIH's growth has stemmed from the congressional
penchant for diseases-of-the-month, and the shrewd assessment of

the medical research establishment and its patrons that it would be easier to get money for tragic diseases, dramatized by real-life heart-wrenching cases, than for basic research identified as such.

The first institute dedicated to a specific disease was the National Cancer Institute, established in 1937. From an initial appropriation of $400,000, its budget grew to $19 million in 1950. With the passage of the National Cancer Act in 1971, huge new resources were pumped into cancer research; the Cancer Institute's budget rocketed to $1.2 billion in 1984.

The major steps in the development of NIH can be traced to mission-oriented institutes: among them, the National Heart, Lung and Blood Institute, the National Eye Institute, and the National Institutes of Dental Research; Mental Health; Neurological and Communicative Disorders and Stroke; Arthritis, Diabetes, Digestive, and Kidney Diseases; Allergy and Infectious Diseases; Child Health and Human Development; Alcohol Abuse and Alcoholism; and Drug Abuse.

By the late 1970s the federal government was funding 90 percent of the basic biomedical research in America. In response to the sharp increase in medical research funds, the faculties and staffs of medical schools grew dramatically, their energies predominantly devoted to research. Between 1950 and 1960, the number of faculty members and research-bent residencies at hospitals more than doubled, even though the number of medical school graduates increased by only 28 percent. World War II GI Bill education benefits paid for graduate training of doctors to do research at hospitals. The postwar expansion of the Veterans Administration hospital system and the VA's search for ways to treat difficult war casualties required many hospitals to establish links with medical schools—and what better way than to give them research funds?

There was serious talk of national health insurance immediately after World War II; spurred by the actions of our ally Great Britain and the advocacy of our feisty president Harry S Truman. The voluntary hospital system in Great Britain had, in effect, been nationalized to deal with the heavy war casualties, and virtually every doctor and nurse was in the British armed forces. So it was a relatively easy step for a socialist government to formalize and perpetuate the situation by taking over the hospitals it was operating and putting doctors and nurses on salary in the National Health Service.

But the United States was not Britain. Our country was relatively unscathed by the war, and the medical profession here was set to resist any such efforts. The doctors had made their sacrifice for the war effort. Now, like most other Americans, they wanted to cash in on the prosperity expected to follow. They were particularly heartened by the money available to pay their fees, courtesy of the new insurance plans springing up in the private sector.

The AMA was ready to fight in 1945, when President Truman proposed a sweeping national health insurance program to cover all Americans, even agricultural workers and others not then protected by Social Security. Truman also suggested new government investments to build hospitals, expand the Public Health Service, and support medical research and education.

Truman tried to allay the fears of doctors and hospitals by assuring them that they could choose whatever method they preferred for payment and delivery of health care services. But the AMA was not buying, especially with the widely anticipated Republican administration of Thomas E. Dewey just around the corner. In the upset of the century, Truman was reelected in 1948, despite the almost fanatical opposition of doctors. In 1949 and 1950 the AMA spent an unprecedented $2.8 million in a massive public relations campaign that effectively branded Truman's national health insurance proposal as socialized medicine, even as part of a Communist plot.

Truman's national health proposal was politically discredited, but Congress did adopt some of his other ideas. In 1946 Congress passed the Hill-Burton program to build hospitals, particularly to increase the number of beds in poor states. By the time the law expired in 1978, the program had used $4.4 billion in federal money as leverage to get state and local governments to ante an additional $9.1 billion. These funds built 500,000 beds, almost half the hospital beds in use in 1985.

In the 1950s health care costs began their relentless rise. The price of hospital care doubled during this decade, from an average of $16 per day in 1950 to $32 per day in 1960. With rising costs and the emergence of an older population as life expectancy inched over sixty-five came pressure from the elderly—and their working children—for some form of government health insurance. Congress responded in 1960 with a program to finance state efforts to help the elderly, sponsored by Senator Robert Kerr of Oklahoma and Congressman Wilbur Mills of Arkansas, then chairman of the House Ways and Means Committee.

Under the Kerr-Mills legislation, the federal government provided states with 50 to 80 percent of the funds they spent for medical assistance to the aged. The poorest states received the highest federal match. Beneficiaries were limited to those in severe financial need. States were free to provide a full range of benefits, from hospital, surgical, and physician care to drugs and false teeth. But by 1963 only thirty-two of the fifty states had established programs, and of these, five large industrial states (New York, California, Massachusetts, Michigan, and Pennsylvania), with only 32 percent of the population over sixty-five, were receiving 90 percent of the funds.

John Kennedy had made health insurance for the elderly a major issue during his 1960 campaign for the presidency. He had proposed it as part of his 1961 legislative program, but like many of his other recommendations to Congress, this one was stymied by a coalition of Republicans and Southern Democrats. It was President Lyndon Johnson who would end the toe-dipping and plunge the federal government into the deep waters of America's health care system.

On assuming the presidency, Johnson turned his legislative genius on the Congress and the American Medical and Hospital associations. Johnson cited Medicare as a major priority in his first speech to Congress, and followed up with a special health message to Congress in early 1964. His commitment to the legislation was total: "We are going to fight for medical care for the aged as long as we have breath in our bodies."

The pending Democratic proposals would have provided only hospital benefits for the aged. Although Johnson wanted more—the focus of his attention was access to a wide range of health care, first for the elderly, eventually for the poor as well—he recognized that to overcome the intransigence of the doctors, hospitals, insurance companies, and their allies, like the Chamber of Commerce and the National Association of Manufacturers, he would have to accept certain compromises. Some had already been made during the long legislative history of the Medicare legislation and were incorporated in his proposals, such as the provisions assuring that hospitals would be paid their "reasonable cost" of providing service to the elderly. Johnson's inclusion of these concessions defused the American Hospital Association's opposition and that of Blue Cross and some commercial insurance companies.

Under intense pressure from Johnson, the Senate Finance Committee held public hearings on Medicare in August 1964. The committee refused to report out a bill, but Johnson and his supporters in the Senate had enough votes to attach Medicare to a bill providing for increased Social Security benefits that had passed the House. Despite strong election-year pressures for the Senate to abandon the Medicare amendment in conference and let the Social Security benefits increase go into effect, Johnson refused to yield on the issue and the bill died in conference. During the conference, House Ways and Means chairman Wilbur Mills promised to give Medicare first priority in the next session. A few weeks later, when Lyndon Johnson brought a two-to-one Democratic majority into the House on his coattails, Mills was ready to act.

After two months of hearings, Mills astutely proposed combining the Democrats' hospitalization-insurance bill for the elderly with a Republican alternative that would create a voluntary program of surgical/medical insurance for them, to be paid through individual premiums and general revenues. In addition, he suggested changing eligibility for the Kerr-Mills program to include most people on welfare and the medically indigent without regard to age, the proposal that would be called Medicaid. President Johnson quickly endorsed Mills's approach.

There was a price to be paid, however. In addition to acceding to the hospitals' demands for reimbursement of their reasonable costs, the legislation provided that these programs would pay physicians fees that were "reasonable," "customary," and in line with those "prevailing" in their community. While cost-based reimbursement was widely used in the hospital industry at the time, insurers did not commonly pay physicians according to their "customary" fees in the mid-1960s. Nevertheless, Johnson accepted this system to blunt AMA claims that government would control doctors' fees. Medicare's adoption of this system had the effect of bringing it into wide use among Blue Shield and commercial insurers, something the medical profession had been trying unsuccessfully to peddle for years. As a result, physicians would gain even greater power to charge what the traffic would bear.

Johnson agreed because his focus was almost entirely on access, rarely on cost. Sitting in Johnson's small green hideaway office one day, White House and HEW lobbyists Larry O'Brien and Wilbur Cohen (later to become Secretary of HEW) responded to Johnson's demand that they move the Medicare bill out of committee. "It'll cost a half-billion dollars to make the changes in reimbursement standards to get the bill out of the Senate Finance Committee," Cohen said.

"Five hundred million. Is that all?" Johnson exclaimed with a wave of his big hand. "Do it. Move that damn bill out now, before we lose it."

A "compromise" was born. It went beyond Medicare paying hospitals on the basis of what their services cost, and doctors their reasonable, customary, and prevailing fees. To keep big government out of the practice of medicine, the legislation also turned over to insurance companies the tasks of paying and auditing doctors and hospitals. And it gave the hospitals the right to pick which insurance companies they wanted to be their auditors! Thus a direct relationship between the providers and the federal government was avoided. Not everyone was happy. But these changes did turn some health insurers into allies of Johnson's proposal and neutralized the resistance of hospitals. They also effectively gutted the arguments of the doctors whose opposition continued; congressmen and senators could now answer their contentions by saying, "You're free of government interference, even on your fees, and a lot of your nonpaying patients will now be sources of income to you."

So Medicare and Medicaid came out of their legislative birth pains in 1965.

We in the Johnson administration did not stop with these programs. Anticipating sharply increased demand for health care services, we pushed through Congress laws to train more doctors and nurses, build more hospitals, and set up community health centers. The assumption was that we were playing by traditional economic rules: the more doctors and hospitals, the more competition, the more efficient and less costly the services.

By 1967 and 1968 we realized how misguided this assumption was. The rise of health care costs was accelerating dramatically. In 1968 I helped draft the President's special message to Congress on Health in America. In that message, Johnson sounded the alarm on inflation in the health care system and cited three "major deficiencies" to be corrected:

- the tilt of insurance plans that "encourage doctors and patients to choose hospitalization"
- the fee-for-service system with "no strong economic incentives to encourage [doctors] to avoid providing care that is unnecessary"
- the fact that "hospitals charge on a cost basis, which places no penalty on inefficient operations"

President Johnson requested authority from the Congress to "employ new methods of payment as they prove effective in providing high quality medical care more efficiently and at lower cost." He warned that unless the nation restrained hospital costs, its health bill could reach $100 billion by 1975, and the cost of medical care for a typical American family would double in seven years.

Newspapers and leaders on Capitol Hill challenged Johnson's numbers and dismissed his words as hyperbole aimed at getting his program passed. Congress failed to act, acceding to do-nothing pressures from the American Medical and Hospital associations.

As it turned out, Johnson's numbers weren't right. By 1975 America's health care bill actually hit $133 billion. And the cost of medical care for an American family did not double in seven years, it doubled in less than six.

The rush of federal dollars to treat patients and increase the number of doctors was accompanied by a boost of funds for research on sophisticated medical techniques. During the 1960s, the federal medical research budget grew from $200 million to $1 billion. In 1965 Johnson pressed for and got Congress to pass the Heart Disease, Cancer, and Stroke bill, which created regional medical centers to provide sophisticated hospital care in every section of the country. The expansion of NIH and the creation of these centers increased the richness and intensity of medical care provided in hospitals across America.

The prevailing attitude was: if such care is far more expensive, so be it. Medicare was picking up the tab for the elderly and big business had agreed to pay the bill for its employees, so plenty of money was available. The vicious circle kept spiraling costs upward with each turn: research funds created a demand for more specialized researchers and scientists, who created new demands for more research funds to support their work, and their spectacular discoveries made the American people willing to pay for more research and to train more specialists. After all, in less than two decades, this investment in research had produced vital-organ transplants, psychiatric and anticancer drugs, electric-shock therapy to revive hearts that had stopped beating, surgical operations that reattached partially severed fingers, hands, and arms, psychosurgery that altered the mind, stunning advances in fetal medicine and the treatment of premature babies, and the ability to extend life for thousands who would have died of heart disease, cancer, stroke, or respiratory complications just a decade earlier.

Nowhere does the good news/bad news nature of the health care problem come into sharper focus than in the experience of the federal government. Medicare, Medicaid, and the research complex have led the way to a healthier nation, sharply increasing life expectancy and the quality of life for senior citizens and significantly improving the health of the poor. At the same time, federal adoption of the cost-based, fee-for-service reimbursement system became a blank check for American hospitals and doctors, and they didn't hesitate to draw on the account. The volume of hospital services reimbursed on a cost or cost-plus basis rose 75 percent owing to Medicare and Medicaid. The rate of increase in hospital spending, which had averaged 8.8 percent between 1960 and 1965, almost doubled, approaching an average annual increase of

15 percent from 1965 to 1970. Sharp rises occurred in hospital staffing, wages, and purchases of new equipment and supplies. Doctors' fees rose rapidly and physicians enriched the treatment of many patients far beyond what was medically appropriate.

The enrichment of care and proliferation of tests have not only directly increased health care costs, they have also set standards by which judges and juries determine whether doctors and hospitals are negligent in treating patients entrusted to their care.

A series of late-nineteenth-century court decisions held that a physician need only meet the standard of care of the local community in which he practiced to avoid liability for malpractice. But scientific invention, medical technology, specialization, Medicare and Medicaid, and the Great Society's regional heart, cancer, and stroke centers nationalized the standard of care for physicians. Batteries of diagnostic tests became routine procedure just to meet those standards.

In the first part of the twentieth century, physicians in a community refused to testify against one another. They organized malpractice funds for legal defenses. Their early success—in its first twenty years of existence, the Washington State medical society won every malpractice case it defended—assured low insurance rates. But as malpractice standards were nationalized, patients' attorneys became more aggressive. Eventually they broke down the physicians' self-protection code, and malpractice suits became forums for determining whether doctors and hospitals had performed every conceivable test available for diagnosing and treating the patient's illness. Too often, failure to perform one test or another was found to be negligent. Once negligence was established by lawyers and judges, juries were given carte blanche to set whopping judgments.

This turn of events gave a two-rocket boost to health care costs. First, in attempting to forestall lawsuits, doctors and hospitals felt compelled to run one test after another, especially since they weren't paying for them. Second, malpractice insurance premiums soared, in 1984 costing doctors $2 billion, and hospitals at least another $1.5 billion.

*   *   *

The health care system did not become bloated by defying the laws of economics. Quite the contrary, everyone in it has acted exactly as the classical economists say they should have, in response to the economic incentives they've faced.

By the early 1980s, virtually all hospitals were reimbursed for their charges on a cost basis, or in the case of for-profit hospitals, a cost-plus basis. Thus, the more they spent, the more they received. Virtually all doctors were paid on a fee-for-service basis. Thus, the more services they performed, the more money they made. Moreover, the patient had no reason to think he was paying these bills. By 1983 more than 90 percent of the hospital bills in America and more than 70 percent of the doctors' bills were paid by government programs like Medicare and Medicaid, private insurers, and the Blues. The health care payment and delivery system had obliterated the tension between buyer and seller that promotes efficiency and cost consciousness.

When an American buys an automobile, he or she chooses a dealer, negotiates about model, price, terms of payment, optional equipment, color, trim, Then the buyer picks the car he or she wants and pays for it. But no one enters a hospital and says, "I would like an appendectomy today," or "I would like a hysterectomy tomorrow." Where hospitalization is involved, the patient doesn't even choose the surgeon or specialist; the family physician does. That surgeon or specialist prescribes the medical procedure and selects the hospital at which it will be performed. Knowing he is not likely to be sued for an extra test—and since he is not paying for them—he has every incentive to run lots of tests. In a cost-based payment system so does the hospital, since its charges for tests help pay for the expensive equipment used to conduct them.

Americans have gotten more tests, seen more physicians, spent more time in hospitals for minor medical procedures, taken more drugs, had more medical examinations, and been subjected to more unnecessary surgery than any other people in the world. And it has all seemed free. In the 1930s, when Americans paid more than 90 percent of their medical bills, it was common for mothers to tell their children to put on their coats in the winter and dry themselves off after their baths, because "we can't afford the doctor's bills if you get sick." Fifty years later, this reason is rarely given, because most Americans have no sense of paying their medical bills.

In a rich system of early-dollar coverage, unlimited choices, and full benefits, having a Blue Cross, commercial health insurance, or Medicare card became like having a credit card to use at restaurants—and never getting a bill. We'd all order caviar, lobster, steak, and Dom Perignon if we had such a credit card. That's the only food and champagne the restaurant would stock. There would be no more crowded tables. The owner would not have to worry about renting unnecessary space, or the cost of linens on empty tables. He would have no concern about moving out the first sitting and turning the tables over twice each evening. Several waiters would hover over each table—one to serve, another to mix the salad, a third to filet the fish, and a fourth whose specialty was whipping the zabaglione.

The health insurance card that let us enter the third-party, fee-for-service, cost-plus health care reimbursement system provided only the illusion of a free lunch. In reality, we have all paid for this meal. And what we've paid has created a health industry colossus.

Chapter 4

THE HEALTH INDUSTRY COLOSSUS

Health has become one of America's biggest businesses. It is the nation's second-largest employer, after education, and third-largest industry in consumer spending, behind only food and housing.

The health industry's piece of the gross national product in 1984 was $387 billion, 10.6 percent. That means Americans broke the billion-dollar-a-day barrier in money they spent on health care in 1984. If the health industry's appetite for our funds continues to grow as it has in the past, health care will set its sights on 15 percent of our gross national product in the early 1990s. At the pace we're going, each man, woman, and child in America will have a $2,600 health care bill in 1990—two-and-one-half times their 1980 share.

The numbers are so big we tend to lose perspective. We pay for health care in everything we purchase. More than one cent of every first-class postage stamp we buy goes to pay for health care for postal workers, their dependents, and retirees, a bill that's been rising at 17 percent a year. Some 15 cents of every federal tax dollar went to the health industry in 1984. For years, government health programs—not defense or Social Security—have been the fastest-rising segment of the federal budget. For millions of workers, the cost of health insurance premiums and health care, not income taxes, has been the major cause of the rapidly widening gap between total compensation and cash taken home. The fastest-

rising cost of doing business has been health care and health insurance premiums, not labor or raw materials.

In 1979 the cost of being born ranged from $1,200 to $2,000 for
a four-day stay in an American hospital; by 1984 the range was
from $1,850 to $2,700 for a three-day stay. The cost of dying has
gone up even faster. Over the same five-year period, Medicare
costs for each dying patient have more than doubled.

We pay more for health care than for chrome or upholstered
bucket seats when we buy a car. In 1984 the auto industry had to
sell at least 500,000 cars and trucks just to pay its health care bills.
For each $500 day a patient spends in the hospital, some $30 of
the bill goes to pay health benefits for hospital employees. Three
cents of the cost of each fast-food hamburger we buy goes to the
health industry. A new automobile tire costing $57 includes $2 for
health care; a $200 airline ticket, $4. Health benefits for active and
retired employees account for $60 of the cost of every metric ton
of aluminum ALCOA produces.

Health costs are a large part of the reason why American steel
can't compete with foreign steel. The United States spent $1,580
per person on health care in 1984—far more than the next highest
outlay, West Germany's $900 per person, three times more than
Japan's $500, and four times Great Britain's $400. Yet, in each of
those nations, health care is sophisticated and modern. Life expectancy is just as high as in the United States and infant mortality is
lower.

In 1984 the unfunded costs for American companies to fulfill
their commitments to provide health care to retirees so overshad-
owed their unfunded pension obligations that the Financial Accounting Standards Board, which establishes the rules followed by
all certified public accountants, began to nudge corporate
America to bring them out of the closet.

The American health care system has grown faster than Jack's
beanstalk. Over the twenty-year period from 1965 through 1984
health care costs rocketed tenfold; hospital bills and physicians'
fees jumped even faster. Over the same period, the consumer price
index also rose, but at less than one-third the breakneck pace of
health care spending. Even with inflation dropping to 4.3 percent

in 1984, payments for physicians' services were up 7 percent and hospital charges up 8.6 percent, double the overall inflation rate.

Where did we Americans spend our money on health care in 1984? We paid some $158 billion to hospitals, almost half of the total. Physicians took $75 billion, about 20 percent. Dentists got $25 billion, some 6 percent. We put $32 billion into nursing homes, some 8 percent. For over-the-counter and prescription drugs, we paid $23 billion. Medical sundries, like iodine and bandages, cost us $3 billion. We also paid:

- $9 billion for professional services from providers other than physicians and dentists, such as those we received from optometrists, podiatrists, and home health agencies
- $7 billion for eyeglasses and appliances like walkers and wheelchairs
- $9 billion for on-the-job health care, school health services, and ambulances
- $11 billion for government public health activities, like immunization programs for flu and children's diseases
- $9 billion to build new health care facilities
- $19 billion to administer health insurance programs

There's something we didn't pay much for. Not nearly enough was spent for health promotion and disease prevention. Less than 1 percent of the federal government's $112 billion health care budget went to keep us away from doctors and dentists, and out of hospitals.

The health care industry employed more than 7 million people in 1984, about 1 out of every 14 working Americans. There are some 500,000 physicians and 1.8 million nurses. Almost 140,000 dentists use 400,000 dental technicians and other office assistants. America's 40,000 pharmacists provide jobs for scores of thousands of assistants.

The health care professionals emerge from an expensive educational system. There are 143 schools of medicine and osteopathy (a training that places special emphasis on the relationship of the muscle and bone systems to all other body systems), 60 schools of dentistry, 72 schools of pharmacy, and some 1,500 programs in colleges and hospitals that train registered nurses.

Between 1972 and 1982, almost one of every seven new jobs was in the health industry. In 1982, while private employment dropped 2 percent, health industry employment rose 4.5 percent. In 1984, though the rate of expansion of health employment slowed, the unemployment rate was only 4.3 percent, compared with the 7.5 percent national rate. While hospital employment actually declined that year, more than 100,000 new jobs were added to other health enterprises. Moreover, employment growth in the health care industry is expected to continue to outpace that in the overall economy, even with a continued decline in hospital employment. By 1995 another 3.35 million persons will be employed, a nearly 50 percent jump.

About 6,900 hospitals in the United States maintain 1.3 million beds. The total number of hospital beds has not changed greatly since the early 1970s, although the portion operated for a profit has increased. If the number of hospital beds has held still for a decade, the number of nursing-home beds has been on a relentless climb. By 1980 America had more nursing home beds than hospital beds, and that spread is expected to widen.

Home health care—providing nursing services in the home, particularly for treatment of chronic illness and the elderly, diagnostic tests and physical therapy—is one of the newest businesses in the industry. In 1980 Congress relaxed restrictions on Medicare reimbursement of home health care costs, and allowed for-profit firms to participate. Over the next three years, the number of for-profit companies in the home health care business more than doubled. Home health care became the most rapidly growing part of the Medicare budget, climbing from $750 million in 1980 to $1.8 billion in 1984. Medicaid paid another $600 million in home health benefits that year. At least a dozen major commercial insurers offer home health care coverage as part of their group policies. As a result, total spending on home health services is predicted to shoot as high as $9 billion by 1986. Home health care is increasing in sophistication, to include services like kidney dialysis and intravenous feeding.

Medical equipment, like pharmaceuticals, has become a major segment of the health care colossus. In 1984 medical equipment manufacturers sold more than $16 billion of their products to doctors, dentists, hospitals, nursing homes, and, largely at the urging of doctors, individual patients. These manufacturers employ 184,-000 people at their 2,600 plants.

Health insurance is the paper workhorse of America's health care industry. In 1984 the health insurance industry wrote group or individual policies with widely varying coverage for some 175 million Americans. More than 1,000 commercial insurance companies and 95 Blue Cross and Blue Shield plans sell and administer these policies.

In 1984 the commercial companies, Blues, health maintenance organizations (HMOs), and corporate and union self-administered plans collected about $120 billion in health insurance premiums. Employers pick up almost 80 percent of that tab for premiums for their employees. The rise in premiums has been as persistent as the rise in the health care costs they have fed and mimicked—an average increase of 14 percent year in and year out for thirty-five years, since 1950.

Commercial insurers and the Blues take the lion's share of our premiums, about $92 billion. Three hundred and thirty-five HMOs provide whatever health care is needed for a prearranged annual payment. If hospitalization is included in the set HMO annual fee, there is usually no additional charge based on length of stay or intensity of care. Americans paid more than $7 billion to HMOs in 1984, again most of it coming from employers for employees. Commercial insurers and Blues have begun to set up their own HMOs.

The largest single customer of the health care industry is the federal government. In 1984 Uncle Sam paid about $112 billion for health care—picking up bills for everything from Medicare and Medicaid ($85 billion) to vaccines for childhood immunization, rehabilitation, veterans' hospitals, care for the military and their dependents, and basic research at the National Institutes of Health in Bethesda, Maryland. Medicare and Medicaid alone paid 29 cents of each of the $342 billion spent in the United States on personal health care, the services provided directly to individuals, as distinguished from money for construction, research, public health, and administering health insurance. State and local governments are also big customers of the health care industry, paying $50 billion for health care in 1984.

America spends more on health research alone than many nations of the world can claim as their entire gross national product. In 1984 the nation's total investment in research was about $11 billion, with the federal government footing just over half of the research bill. Business pays most of the rest, largely focused on commercially attractive results, like discovering new drugs, developing high-technology equipment, and putting genes to work to diagnose, prevent, and cure disease.

Any industry that gobbles up more than 10 percent of our gross national product will spawn its share of parasites and hangers-on. You can now charge your medical bills on your American Express, Visa, or MasterCard at thousands of doctors' offices, hospitals, and nursing homes throughout the United States. No state legislature can get through a session without being besieged by lobbyists representing doctors, hospitals, health insurers, and public interest groups. In Washington, D.C., the world's mecca for such labors, no less than 300 organizations lobby the Congress, the executive branch, and each other on health industry issues. In 1984 the American Medical Association's political action committee invested $3 million just in congressional candidates. There are hundreds of magazines and scholarly and trade journals published on health issues; columns by doctors, psychologists, and nutritionists in most newspapers; books on health care from every publishing house; hundreds of Wall Street analysts and investment bankers looking for the best stocks and mergers; thousands of accountants and attorneys who help them; thousands more who make their living interpreting and manipulating Medicare regulations to get the most money out of the government for their clients; still other thousands of attorneys who spend their careers suing or defending hospitals, drug companies, and doctors at the medical malpractice bar. The pots of gold on the fringes of the health industry's rainbow are real. Large numbers of American businesses are mining their share, and those who aren't have begun their prospecting.

* * *

Far more troubling than the size of the health care industry is its inefficiency and lack of discipline, which have provided a breeding ground for waste and abuse. A 1984 study sponsored by the Department of Health and Human Services examined Medicare and Medicaid admissions during 1980 at twenty-five carefully selected representative hospitals, urban and rural, in various regions of the country. The study concluded that 19 percent of all admissions were unnecessary or premature, and that 27 percent of the hospital days were completely inappropriate. A 1984 study of sixteen hospitals in Flint, Grand Rapids, and Lansing, Michigan, found that 21 percent of the hospital admissions should never have occurred and that 22 percent of the hospital days were unnecessary. A 1984 General Accounting Office study revealed that more than 30 percent of the patients in Veterans Administration hospitals didn't belong there, including not only those needlessly admitted, but also those admitted too soon, kept too long, or hospitalized for tests that could have been performed in less expensive outpatient settings. Chrysler Corporation's detailed examination of its health care system indicated that 25 percent of the hospitalization and treatment of its employees, retirees, and dependents, in and out of hospitals, was unnecessary and inappropriate.

Pause on the implications of these findings. If 25 percent of the health care bill in 1984 was inappropriate—a genteel word to cover everything from honest mistake and inefficiency to bad medicine to deliberate fraud—then Americans unnecessarily spent almost $100 billion dollars in 1984!

In 1978, when I was Secretary of Health, Education, and Welfare, I started using computers as policemen to ferret out fraud and abuse in the Medicare and Medicaid programs. We called the effort Project Integrity. We set up limits in the computers for the performance of twenty-two medical procedures by an individual physician on a single patient. For example, we programmed the computer to spot any doctor who billed for more than one appendectomy on the same patient in the same year, for an abortion after billing for a hysterectomy on the same woman, for more than forty office visits by the same patient in the same year, for more than one tonsillectomy for the same patient, or for more than ten X-rays on the same patient in one year. To catch crooked pharmacists, we selected twenty-six commonly used drugs, like Librium and Valium. The computer cops tagged pharmacists who filled more than 50 Valium prescriptions for the same patient in one year, or two or more prescriptions for the same drug on the same day for a single recipient, and who billed for prescription drugs but actually dispensed over-the-counter items.

In the initial year of Project Integrity, we identified 47,000 physicians and pharmacists who broke the computer limits. Indeed, so many providers ripped off the Medicaid program that we were able to prosecute only the fifty most egregious offenders in each state. Scores of individuals were convicted of criminal activities; hundreds of administrative sanctions, like denial of participation in Medicare or Medicaid programs, were imposed; and millions of dollars were recovered. But the health care system is so undisciplined and susceptible to fraud and abuse that the federal government finds thousands of examples every year. In 1984 federal and state investigators successfully prosecuted 500 health care providers and suppliers, kicked out of Medicare and Medicaid 350, and saved taxpayers more than half a billion dollars. Here are a few examples:

- A physician billed Medicare and Medicaid for hundreds of hospital visits, lab tests, and other procedures that were never performed. He was convicted on 82 counts.
- Another physician claimed he performed a full rectal exam, and reported no abnormalities, on a patient whose rectum had previously been removed surgically. He was suspended from Medicare and Medicaid participation for five years.
- An ambulance company filed $500,000 in false Medicare claims for driving phantom patients for kidney dialysis treatments. The company was suspended for five years.
- A pharmacist billed Medicaid for brand name drugs, dispensed far less expensive generic drugs, and pocketed the difference. He was suspended for six years.
- A therapist charged Medicare for speech therapy for deceased and comatose patients. He was sentenced to three years in prison.

In addition to uncovering rip-offs, federal fraud and abuse investigations have identified numerous instances of leakage in the health care programs: for instance, the lack of controls that has permitted millions of dollars in duplicate payments by Medicare and the Veterans Administration for the same medical services in nursing homes, and has allowed housekeeping services, such as shopping and ironing, to be charged to Medicaid at an estimated $30 million annually.

The private sector has been no more efficient and no less abuse-prone. In my experience with Chrysler, I found waste and abuse at virtually every point we touched the health care system. Similar waste and inefficiency have festered in almost every health benefit program in this country.

Any multibillion-dollar enterprise will have a certain level of fraud and waste, whether it's the defense industry, real estate, or the transportation business. What's been so disturbing about the health care industry has been the absence of checks and balances that normally operate to temper profligacy and cheating: the lack of competition, the elimination of tension between buyer and seller, the ineffectiveness of regulatory controls in the face of a supplier-controlled payment and delivery system.

Perhaps we could tolerate a good measure of abuse and waste if we were otherwise getting our money's worth, if Americans were the healthiest people on earth. While the United States spent $1,580 for each man's, woman's, and child's health care in 1984, Singapore spent less than $200. Yet both countries have the same rate of life expectancy at birth, and Singapore's appears to be rising more rapidly. Singapore's infant mortality is lower than ours. Indeed, seven other nations have infant mortality rates lower than ours.

Nor are we buying a fair health care system. Millions of our citizens still lack adequate health care, and while there have been marked improvements in life expectancy and infant mortality for blacks, there are still gaping disparities between blacks and whites with respect to life expectancy and the health status of men and babies. Nor is more money buying more health insurance for all our citizens. The Urban Institute estimates that from 1979 to 1983 the number of Americans under sixty-five without health insurance coverage went from 29 million to 33 million. In a 1984 study, the Department of Health and Human Services concluded that 35 million Americans had no health insurance for at least part of the year, and another 16 million had inadequate coverage. If we could save just 10 percent in health care costs by eliminating waste and inefficiency—a distinctly modest goal—that $40 billion would be more than enough to provide essential care to those millions of our citizens who at best get catch-as-catch-can care from hospital emergency rooms willing to treat them, or at worst, and far too often, get no care at all.

America is awakening to the health care cost crisis it faces, and none too soon. For too long in the health care area, we have let tomorrow take care of itself because the troubles of today appeared to be elsewhere. But in 1986 and beyond, whether a president and Congress work on the federal deficit, or a corporate chief executive tries to reduce the cost of doing business, or a husband and wife struggle to manage the family budget, health care costs loom among the top financial problems they—and hence our nation—face.

There are signs that our awakening to these problems can lead to results, particularly in the gold-plated hospital sector. But transforming the American way of health is no task for the timid. It will demand imagination, persistence, and courage. One critical challenge is to convince the doctors that we are serious about making fundamental changes in the system, to make it clear to them that we want results.

Chapter 5

THE MEDICINE MEN

The doctors are the medicine men and women of 1980s America. They are the powerful high priests of the health care industry. They hold the keys that let us into the health care system, and almost all of us stay until they let us out, especially when they put us into one of their hospitals. Without them we can't get tranquilizers to calm our nerves, potent drugs to ease our pain, pills to relieve our hypertension, or radiation treatment to arrest our cancer.

For the $75 billion we paid physicians in 1984, they told us to pay another $200 billion to hospitals for inpatient care, and to laboratories and pharmacies, pathologists and nurses, for all sorts of tests of our blood, sputum, urine, and other body solids and liquids, for X-rays, scans, and photographs of our insides, for millions of enemas, stress tests, and electrocardiograms, and for billions of prescription pills.

Doctors work hard, often with a selfless dedication that jeopardizes their own health, at what our society trains and pays them to do. Researchers produce medical miracles. Specialists perform the most delicate surgery on the heart and brain. Hospital-based physicians keep us alive under the most extraordinary circumstances, with machines that clean our blood and breathe for us. Family doctors treat and soothe us with all sorts of drugs that we've come to expect from them. Doctors try their best to find out what's wrong with us and then to cure our illness and repair our bodies.

America's 500,000 physicians constitute less than 7 percent of the people who work in the health care industry. But they influence just about every aspect of it.

Each year, these physicians see 75 percent of the American people in more than 1.3 billion office or hospital visits. That's almost six visits for each man, woman, and child in the country. Doctors recommend almost 40 million hospital admissions, resulting in 375 million patient-days of service. They write a billion and a half prescriptions just for patients not in the hospital, almost seven for each man, woman, and child. When we add together what we pay doctors and the cost of what they prescribe for us in tests, pills, appliances, surgery, and other medical treatment, that accounts for more than 70 percent of all health care costs.

Who are these high priests of American medicine? How well trained are they for the power they exercise over our lives and our pocketbooks? Are they too many or too few? How necessary are they to our good health? Are they overpaid? Do they work too hard? Do we accord them too much deference? Could we run the health care system without them?

WHAT THE MEDICAL SCHOOLS DON'T TEACH

To become a medicine man or woman in the 1980s, a student has to suffer through grueling years of training crammed with thousands of scientific facts to be memorized; attend hundreds of hours of lectures by faculty members, many of whom prefer research or patient care to teaching; and spend night upon night with little or no sleep.

Virtually all the frenetic scheduling and detailed drudgery of the medical school years and hospital internships and residencies is designed to teach students how to treat the sick. Brilliant, high-fee, prestigious physician-professors encourage specialization. So "my son the doctor" has given way to "my son the cardiologist," "my son the ophthalmologist," "my daughter the brain surgeon." Finding courses on cost consciousness, health promotion, or disease prevention in medical schools is about as hard as finding a subway car without graffiti in New York.

Physicians must play a central role in any serious effort to get the American people to take care of themselves. Yet virtually no clinical time is spent on disease prevention or health promotion in our fledgling doctors' internships and residencies. In 1984 those topics were allocated a mere 1.5 percent of the teaching time in America's medical schools, as the Harvard University president's annual report disclosed. Health promotion and disease prevention are not, after all, what patients pay the doctor for, despite the fact that changes in life-style—such as quitting smoking, drinking alcohol in moderation, getting enough exercise and sleep, handling stress, eating properly—can cut illness in half in the United States.

Addiction is one of America's overarching health problems, yet it's hard to find out much about it in medical school classrooms. Fifty million Americans are hooked on cigarettes, 3.5 million of them under the age of 17; 13 million are addicted to alcohol or abuse it; millions more are addicted to heroin, cocaine, marijuana, tranquilizers, barbiturates, sedatives, and a variety of other pills.

Take two of addiction's most pernicious forms: alcohol abuse and cigarette smoking.

Alcoholism and alcohol abuse together are the number-four disease in America, right behind the big three of heart and circulatory diseases, cancer, and respiratory diseases. If current trends persist, alcoholism and alcohol abuse will outpace the others at the turn of the century. In most large cities, up to 40 percent of hospital emergency-room admissions and 25 percent of inpatient admissions are alcohol-related. Alcoholism has been an enigma for medical research, but we know two things for sure: prevention is the most effective cure, and the earlier alcohol abuse is detected, the greater the likelihood of arresting the disease. Yet most medical schools devote less than 1 percent of classroom time to prevention and treatment of alcoholism over the four-year curriculum, and medical training tends to neglect teaching doctors how to spot alcohol abusers.

Each year, cigarette smoking kills some 360,000 Americans, through cardiovascular disease (170,000), cancer (130,000), and chronic respiratory diseases (60,000), and maims and disables hundreds of thousands more. Seventy percent of the mothers whose babies die from sudden infant death syndrome—the single greatest cause of infant death—are cigarette smokers. Giving up cigarettes

FOODS THAT CAUSE PAIN

Headache Triggers

Alcohol

Artificial Sweetener

Aspartame

Baked Goods

Caffeine

Cheese

Chocolate

Citrus Fruits

Containing Yeast

Cured Meats

Monosodium Glutamate

Nuts

Sauerkraut

Yogurt

Top Arthritis Triggers

(Listed from most common to least common)

1. Corn
2. Wheat
3. Pork
4. Oranges
5. Milk
6. Oats
7. Rye
8. Eggs
9. Beef
10. Coffee
11. Malt
12. Cheese
13. Grapefruit
14. Tomato
15. Peanuts
16. Sugar
17. Butter
18. Lamb
19. Lemon
20. Soybeans

To test a food you suspect may be causing your problems:

Eliminate the food from your diet for one week. If your symptoms subside, you may have identified one of your food triggers. You can double-check by reintroducing the suspect food into your diet to see if your symptoms return.

Discover more surprising health dangers and cures in

NATURAL MEDICINES AND CURES YOUR DOCTOR NEVER TELLS YOU ABOUT

FOODS THAT EASE PAIN

More and more scientific research known for a long time. The same foods supports what home healers have that please your palate can sometimes food remedies for relieving arthritis and put a stop to your pain.

Arthritis and Headache Pain

Ginger is one of the most effective food remedies for relieving arthritis and headache pain.

To relieve arthritis pain:
- Take about 1/3 teaspoon three times a day. Dissolve in liquid or mix with food — straight ginger can burn your mouth.

To relieve headache pain:
- At the first sign of a headache, mix 1/3 teaspoon powdered ginger in a glass of water and drink. You can also relieve headaches by rubbing a ginger paste on your forehead.

Migraine Headache Pain
Peppermint Tea works wonders.
1. Boil one pint of water.
2. Remove from heat and add two tablespoons of fresh or dried peppermint leaves.
3. Cover mixture and let steep for two minutes, strain.
   Drink 1-2 cups of tea.

Long-Term Headache Cure
Including fish in your diet can help lessen the frequency of migraine headaches. Choose fish such as mackerel, sardines, salmon and tuna.

Pain from Diabetes and Shingles

The active ingredient in red peppers, capsaicin, effectively relieves discomfort caused by these debilitating conditions. Capsaicin is available as a non-prescription cream (under the brand name Zostrix®) and in hot pepper capsules available in herb shops.

C-FVA

is a more effective cure for recurring ulcers than the leading ulcer drug. Yet the medicine men are not trained to prescribe programs to help patients quit smoking, and though they may deliver an occasional admonition against smoking, thousands of them still permit it in their waiting rooms.

When we consider the abuse of substances of all kinds—alcohol, cigarettes, heroin, cocaine, marijuana, Librium and Valium, Quaaludes, sedatives, barbiturates, and other drugs—we can see why addiction tops America's health problems. Aside from the small amount of attention to alcoholism, however, many medical schools devote no teaching time specifically to substance abuse, or give this pressing health problem only a few lectures over the four-year period.

Nutrition is central to America's health. In terms of the illnesses that plague us, to a significant degree we are what we eat. The National Academy of Sciences links our eating habits to six of the ten leading causes of death—heart disease, stroke, cancer, diabetes, arteriosclerosis, and cirrhosis of the liver. What, and how much, we put into our stomachs can markedly increase or decrease the chance of a serious or fatal heart attack. Obesity afflicts 34 million Americans. Yet only 23 of 127 American medical schools require students to take a course in nutrition. And these courses are often off the mark, dealing more with chemistry than with practical information about everyday diets and foods. Even at Harvard Medical School, first-year students had to stage an organized campaign in 1983 and 1984 to get a nutrition course, because the subject had not been scheduled for introduction into the curriculum until 1985. One University of California medical school did not institute a preventive medicine curriculum, underlining nutrition, until its students demanded one. In 1985, the National Academy of Sciences urged that 25 to 30 hours of teaching be devoted to nutrition, but few schools place anything like the proper emphasis on the entire subject.

Exercise is also essential for good health. By and large American medical education—which takes its own toll on the exercise habits of its students, interns, and residents—has tended to look down on exercise programs as morning television pop health. Yet proper exercise at all ages is an element of good health, and sophisticated cardiologists are even writing out prescriptions for exercise programs for heart-attack victims, instead of just ordering up pills.

The typical family doctor has a hundred opportunities each week to talk to patients who need help because of behavioral risk factors, such as obesity, insufficient exercise, smoking, excessive alcohol consumption, or drug abuse. How many of these opportunities is he trained or paid to use?

Gerontology is another field neglected by medical schools. By the early 1980s, 60 percent of doctors' work was with elderly Americans, our fastest-growing population group. Yet physicians receive precious little training in treating their physical and psychological problems. No American medical school even had a department of geriatrics until 1983, when Mount Sinai in New York City began one. At Mount Sinai, every senior medical student must take four weeks of geriatric training, including two weeks of clinical work at a nursing home. For the most part, however, medical schools offer only short elective courses in geriatrics, which have low enrollments because students are not encouraged to take them.

Psychology also gets short shrift from medical education. Somewhere between 30 and 50 percent of all patients who see a family doctor have no physical or biomedical ailment. Moreover, for whatever reason—guilt, embarrassment, lack of trust—patients do not reveal up to one-half of their prior maladies and hospitalizations. Yet primary-care physicians are rarely trained in psychology. They're often unable to spot mental or emotional problems or detect a patient's equivocation. The blame rests directly on the teaching doctors of the medical profession who, as Harvard president Derek Bok points out, exude an attitude of such disdain about behavioral subjects (and ethics) that "in an environment dominated by science and research, small wonder that only three or four students in each [Harvard] class of 165 actually choose to take more than the bare minimum of these subjects."

Health care costs merit far more attention in the medical school curriculum. Physician professors, who themselves have paid insufficient attention to spiraling medical bills, make little effort to give their students some sense of the need to be cost-conscious and efficient. In 1984, only four schools required courses in cost containment; only seventeen even had electives in the field; others either ignore the problem or claim to include some material on cost consciousness in other courses. Although Harvard Medical School students and faculty have long identified "seeking lower cost solutions to clinical problems" as an area most demanding greater emphasis, only in 1984 did the faculty begin to assemble a sensible curriculum. The need is great: most doctors don't know, within 25 percent, the cost of laboratory tests they prescribe. Few care. And some proclaim with pride that they never consider cost in treating a patient.

As part of its 1983 report on medical education and the needs of our people, the Institute of Medicine of the National Academy of Sciences noted that disease-prevention and health-promotion training of physicians can "provide an integrating principle for medical education and clinical practice." The institute's report attributed many treatment failures to lack of understanding of health promotion:

> Prevention-oriented medical education (and subsequent practice) is not only a body of knowledge and skills, but also a set of attitudes, including an activist stance in encounters with patients for whom prevention measures are appropriate, and a belief in the value of continuity of care. The goal is to identify a patient's potential (preventable) problems as well as current ones.

The medical student's lack of training to carry on the work of health promotion and disease prevention, assess the psychological and behavioral roots of patient distress, and seek cost-effective treatment contributes to his ignorance as a physician about the potential of nonmedical systems to help patients. This ignorance is reinforced by the doctor's economic and professional incentives to keep all treatment in the medical family.

Alcoholism is a case in point. Once it is recognized, we know how to treat alcoholism with a high percentage of success, using mostly nonmedical systems: dry the alcoholic out in a hospital or other acute care facility; then place the patient in a residential controlled-treatment center for a month of intense therapy, and then return the alcoholic to his home. If there is a loving companion—spouse, child, relative, or friend—and if the alcoholic has a job (or task in life) and joins Alcoholics Anonymous, the likelihood of recovery is over 75 percent.

If a physician does not spot alcoholism or alcohol abuse, his lack of training often leads him to the wrong treatment. Normally, the family doctor will urge the patient to stop or reduce his drinking. The accommodating patient will soon tell his doctor that he's nervous. Too frequently, the doctor then prescribes tranquilizers, like Librium or Valium, America's most-abused drugs. Next the alcoholic is likely to report trouble sleeping. Many physicians prescribe a sedative or sleeping pill. Soon the alcoholic patient is drinking again, but this time he also uses his physician-prescribed tranquilizers and barbiturates to relax and sleep. Indeed, so common is this tragic situation that in my visits to alcohol treatment centers across the United States, I rarely found any patient who had abused only alcohol. Most were also on tranquilizers and sleeping pills, and virtually all had started on them courtesy of their doctor.

A critical element here is the reluctance of many doctors to place a patient outside the part of the health care system they control—even when far more efficient treatment of the disease is available there. Once the patient is dried out, a process that is best supervised by a doctor and that takes anywhere from a couple of days to a week, the rest of the treatment is not controlled by the medicine men. Nor should it be. But too many doctors have tried to keep it all in the family, to use pills only they can prescribe, to refer patients only to others with the same credentials.

HOW LITTLE THE MEDICINE MEN KNOW

Don Fredrickson, former head of the National Academy of Sciences Institute of Medicine and Director of the National Institutes of Health while I was Secretary of Health, Education, and Welfare, has presided over and been privy to more medical miracles and inventions than most of his colleagues. In one of our meetings in 1979, we were talking about the medical profession's inability to stem the ravages of Hubert Humphrey's cancer. "You know, Joe," Dr. Fredrickson said, "what's the most important thing for you to know about medicine?"

"What," I asked.

"How little we know," he answered somberly.

We are so inundated with the miracles of modern medicine that we tend to forget how far along this century was before a patient who visited a doctor had a better than fifty-fifty chance of being helped. And then, the help was far more likely to be relief of annoying symptoms than care of the underlying illness or any significant repair beyond what nature itself would accomplish.

Even today, despite the multimillion-dollar array of tools we have placed at the doctor's disposal, the first step—correctly diagnosing the ailment—is no sure bet. And treatments for the same diagnosis vary widely. In a medical system where doctors are paid only when they do something, and patients want something done, uncertainty about diagnosis and treatment makes for all kinds of unnecessary tests and treatments. There is general agreement that surgery is the proper treatment for the repair of an inguinal hernia. But studies spanning the past dozen years show that no such consensus exists with respect to many other common ailments.

Take hemorrhoids that require treatment beyond over-the-counter relief from widely televised drugs. In the five largest hospital service areas in Maine, rates of surgery to remove hemorrhoids varied from half to almost three times the state average in 1973.

Or hysterectomies. In different areas of Maine, the rate varied from 60 to 160 percent of the state average.

Or tonsillitis. In Maine, where you live has determined whether the treatment is to cut your tonsils out or something far less draconian, like antibiotics. Tonsillectomies were performed more than twice as often in the area with the highest rate compared with the lowest.

A 1984 Massachusetts survey of surgery rates revealed even more startling variations. If you lived in Hingham in 1984, you were four times more likely to have your gall bladder removed than if you lived in Holyoke and had the same symptoms. If you want to keep your tonsils and treat the infection with antibiotics, then stay away from Fairhaven, Fitchburg, and Framingham. Residents of those three Massachusetts towns were fifteen times more likely to have tonsillectomies than people living in other Bay State areas. The rate of cesarean section delivery of babies varied from 22 to 48 percent of the births in sixteen Massachusetts communities—rates that many obstetricians consider excessive.

The rates at which doctors send patients to hospitals for minor surgery that they could perform in their offices vary at least as widely, at an unnecessary cost of millions of dollars. Doctors in Framingham and Holliston sent their patients to the hospital for tooth extractions at four times the state average. Eighteen of the 172 Massachusetts communities investigated had hospitalization rates for tooth extraction more than twice the state average. Similar discrepancies in hospitalization rates were revealed for cardiac catheterization across the state.

These studies of disparity in treatment began in 1973. Typical variations uncovered between the lowest and highest surgical rates, if projected nationally in 1984, would have amounted to a cost difference of about $16 billion—almost 10 percent of the nation's hospital bill. And the surveys have repeatedly revealed even greater variations in hospital admission rates for nonsurgical cases, such as gastrointestinal and chronic lung disorders.

Dr. John E. Wennberg, the Dartmouth Medical School professor who originated the investigative technique used in the Massachusetts and Maine investigations (and equally disturbing inquiries in Iowa, Vermont, and Rhode Island, which exposed similarly divergent and erratic medical practices) believes that the variances reveal physician uncertainty about whether to perform numerous common operations, and "the intellectual confusion and chaos that sit at the root of much medical practice." Harvard School of Public Health professor Benjamin A. Barnes, who conducted the Massachusetts study, thinks the most telling conclusion is that "differences exist that do not in any way reflect differences among" residents of the communities investigated. In other words, he added, the differences have no "rational explanation."

These variations may not have a rational explanation in terms of medical practice, but they provide telling insight into the way physicians act in the face of uncertainty. These investigations, conducted by doctors themselves, are of treatments for common, everyday medical diagnoses: tonsillitis, gall bladder problems, hemorrhoids, tooth extractions, arteriosclerosis, and simple pneumonias. In many communities the standard is: when unsure about treatment, put the patient in the hospital and when you can, cut. When there is doubt about diagnosis or a more complex ailment is found, the uncertainty increases, and so does the incentive to do more tests, prescribe more pills, perform more surgery. However well-motivated the physician's urge to do something to help the patient, it costs billions of dollars in unnecessary procedures across the medical care system. In 1984 Dr. Wennberg estimated that adoption of more conservative surgical and medical practice styles by doctors could easily produce a 40 percent reduction in money spent for hospitalization alone—a saving of more than $60 billion in 1984, almost 20 percent of all personal health care expenditures. The former dean of the School of Public Policy, University of California at Berkeley, Aaron Wildavsky, uses the term "Medical Uncertainty Principle" to describe what happens when:

> ... doctor and patient both are uncertain as to what is wrong or what to do about it.... The Medical Uncertainty Principle states that there is always one more thing that might be done—another consultation, a new drug, a different treatment. Uncertainty is resolved by doing more: the patient asks for more, the doctor orders more. The patient's simple rule for resolving uncertainty is to seek care up to the level of his insurance.

THE DOCTORS' ECONOMIC UPSIDE-DOWN CAKE

For most doctors, the bucks are in treatment of disease, not in its prevention or in health promotion.

If your car breaks down or is damaged in an accident, you take it to a dealer or mechanic who tells you what he thinks is wrong and gives you a free estimate of the cost of repair. If your wristwatch slows or stops, you can take it to a jeweler and get a free estimate of what's wrong and how much money you'll have to pay to fix it. The analogy isn't perfect, but if your body doesn't feel right, you have to pay the doctor just to get the estimate. Doctors have established a system in which the only way you can find out whether you need them is to pay them to tell you. So the first ingredient in the economic upside-down cake of physician care is that the supplier decides whether the customer needs supplies.

But there's another important ingredient: the physician supplier also decides just what supplies the customer needs—quality, quantity, how long to maintain the flow of supplies, how rich their mix, where the customer should obtain them. To return to the lexicon of medical care, while most doctors discuss options with patients in complex cases, ordinarily the doctor tells the patient what treatment the patient needs, how long the treatment should continue, who should administer the treatment, and in what setting.

The icing on the cake has been the absence of competition among suppliers, and the resulting lack of limits on the amount of services they provide or what they charge.

Are there too many medicine men performing too many medical procedures?

In business—manufacturing and selling cars, television sets, umbrellas, shoes, hats, or balls—the more suppliers, the lower the cost, because competition drives the prices down. In the economic upside-down cake of medicine, however, more doctors do not necessarily mean lower prices. Indeed, in a provider-controlled system, the more doctors, the more medical services; the more surgeons, the more surgery; the more psychiatrists, the more fifty-minute patient hours on couches; the more specialists, the more referrals to specialists.

The big jump in the number of physicians began in the late sixties, prompted by the Great Society health manpower programs to provide enough doctors to satisfy the new demands of senior citizens and poor people for health care. Great Society planners (of whom I was one) believed more doctors would be needed not only to provide services to these newcomers to the health care system, but also to avoid soaring price increases due to sharply increased demand without new suppliers. We were convinced that doctors had kept their numbers down to keep their prices up. So we crafted, and the Congress passed in 1965, a broad package of amendments to the Health Professions Educational Assistance Act to provide funds to encourage medical schools to double—from

8,000 to 16,000—the number of physicians graduating each year. The strenuous opposition of the medical profession confirmed our belief that more physicians would mean more competition and thus hold down doctors' fees.

To ease physicians' and citizens' concern about the federal government getting into curriculum planning—an issue that came up repeatedly during debate on all Great Society education proposals—we suggested a system of capitation payments with virtually no strings. Medical schools would get federal funds based on the number of students: the more students, the more money. We also established grant and loan programs to help students pay tuition, with no limits on the tuition medical schools could charge.

The medical schools responded. We got lots more doctors; by 1979, we were right up to the 16,000 graduates per year we'd hoped for. But we hadn't reckoned on the impact of physician control of prices and services, or on the explosion of specialization. The combined force of both those elements was ferocious: more doctors meant decidedly higher costs, and more specialists meant a richer mix of medical services, a one-two punch ending with an uppercut that sent the cost of health care through the roof.

In a system where doctors could charge reasonable, customary, and prevailing fees and specialists commanded a premium, doubling the number of physicians more than doubled what they billed, largely as a result of a disproportionate increase in the number of specialists, who got the highest fees. Moreover, because the reasonable, customary, and prevailing fees varied from market to market, physicians in urban centers got more money than those in rural areas, so doctors had an added incentive to cluster in cities.

In 1963 there were 143 physicians for each 100,000 Americans. In 1985 the ratio of physicians to population was 218 for each 100,000. Compare this ratio with that in other medically sophisticated countries to get a sense of America's oversupply. In 1984 the number of physicians reported for each 100,000 people in France was 172; in Great Britain, 154; in Japan, 128. Germany has more physicians per 100,000 population than the United States, but far fewer specialists.

As Secretary of HEW, I was so concerned about the increase in the number of physicians I asked the Graduate Medical Education National Advisory Committee, headed by Dr. Alvin R. Tarlov (then teaching at the University of Chicago's School of Medicine, later to become president of the Kaiser Family Foundation), to look into the problem. Armed with a massive three-year study, the committee sounded the alarm: unchecked, it concluded, the number of physicians would increase to 536,000 (220 per 100,000) by 1990, some 70,000 more than we'll need, and would rise even more sharply thereafter. In 1984 Dr. Tarlov expected that by the year 2000, there would be more than 630,000 doctors (232 per 100,000), some 130,000 more than we'll need.

Even though medical school enrollments are showing some slight decline since 1982, these projections of excess physicians may turn out to be low. They were based on the premise that the maximum number of physicians needed under our current health care system is between 188 and 190 per 100,000 people. If HMOs, preferred providers, and other prepaid plans continue their rapid growth, 120 million Americans (out of an estimated population of 270 million) could be members by the year 2000. Under such plans, fewer doctors are needed, only 106 for each 100,000 people served. Thus, there will be 334 doctors for each 100,000 people among the 150 million Americans not in such plans, an excess far beyond the projections of the 1980 study and the 1984 update by Dr. Tarlov. Moreover, if hospitalization rates and lengths of stay continue to decrease for this group, its need for physicians will approach the low number needed for the HMO population. That will give America a total of more than 300,000 excess doctors in the year 2000.

What do too many physicians mean in terms of costs? In 1984 each new doctor added an estimated $300,000 in additional health care costs. If there had been 130,000 more doctors than we needed in 1984 (as projected for the year 2000), we would have spent an additional $39 billion. If the fee-for-service, third-party reimbursement system based on reasonable, customary, and prevailing fees were not by far the most common method of payment, an excess of doctors might have traditional economic results of increased unemployment and lower prices. In the Netherlands, which has a higher ratio of doctors to population than the United

States, physicians had a 4 percent unemployment rate in 1983 (about a thousand were out of work). Belgium, which also has a higher ratio than the United States, has seen the income of doctors drop sharply since 1980, especially among younger physicians. So if we change the way we have been paying the medicine men, traditional market forces can work to reduce fees in situations of significant oversupply.

It's not simply the number of physicians that spells trouble for the health care system. It's also that they are too specialized and badly dispersed geographically. In 1931, 94 percent of America's doctors were family physicians, delivering primary care to their patients. By 1984 less than 40 percent of our doctors were primary care physicians; the rest were specialists. In France, 60 percent of the physicians are in primary care; in West Germany, 54 percent; in Great Britain, 73 percent. Even the association representing the medical colleges that have trained all these specialists has concluded that at least 50 percent of our doctors should be in primary care.

But the incentives in terms of money and status within (and without) the medical community promote specialization. Most doctors are well paid: in 1984 the average net income for physicians topped $100,000. However, primary care physicians such as family practitioners and general pediatricians, have an average net income of about half, or less than half, of what specialists make. The superspecialists—the coronary bypass surgeons; the heart, cancer, brain, and cataract surgeons—can make ten or more times what a family practitioner does.

The geographic distribution of doctors is also skewed. In 1983 the ratio of physicians to population in urban areas was more than twice what it was in rural areas. In many rural areas there are no physicians at all. The situation has improved since the late 1970s, but physicians remain heavily concentrated in metropolitan areas. There are 610 physicians for each 100,000 people in Manhattan, contrasted with 50 to 70 doctors for each 100,000 residents of upstate New York counties.

The increased supply of physicians may be easing doctor shortages in some areas of the country, but it may also be aggravating the tilt to specialization. In 1960 American towns with a population of 10,000 to 20,000 people were scrapping to get a family physician; less than a third of the towns with a population between 20,000 and 30,000 had a specialist. By the early 1980s, 70 percent of the towns with populations of 10,000 to 20,000 had at least one family practitioner; and more than 70 percent of the towns with populations between 20,000 and 30,000 had five specialists.

The medical schools are beginning to face the oversupply problem. First-year medical school enrollment declined in 1982 for the first time in seventeen years, and in 1984, after three years of declining first-year enrollments, total enrollment in medical schools dropped for the first time in thirty-seven years—a reflection of the schools' concern about physician oversupply and reductions in federal aid. Yet with the doctor's license widely regarded as a ticket to great affluence and prestige, medical schools, despite tuitions averaging $15,000 a year and ranging to more than $25,000, are still oversubscribed.

In addition to the domestic production of doctors, each year 5,000 graduates of foreign medical schools (many of them are Americans) qualify for internship or residency slots in the United States. In 1984 an estimated 12,000 U.S. citizens were studying in medical schools abroad. Here, too, efforts are under way to reduce these numbers, chiefly through stiffer qualifying exams for graduates of foreign medical schools.

Perhaps the most extraordinary thing about the economic upside-down cake physicians have concocted is that we've let them bake it for so long. Listen to Dr. Richard Cabot, Harvard Medical School professor, speaking back in 1938:

> We would never put a judge on the bench under conditions such that he might be influenced by pecuniary considerations. Suppose that if the judge were to hand down one decision he got $5,000, and if he decided the other way he got nothing. But we allow the private practitioner to face this sort of temptation.
>
> The greatest single curse in medicine is the curse of unnecessary operations, and there would be fewer of them, if the doctor got the same salary whether he operated or not.

I am not accusing the medical profession of dishonesty, but I am saying that we should be defended from unfair temptation. I maintain that to have doctors working on salary would be better for doctors as well as for patients.

The point is not that doctors are more or less honest than the rest of us. Rather, the point is that their economic self-interest is served by performing medical services: running batteries of tests to avoid malpractice suits; identifying illnesses to cure, gall bladders and hemorrhoids to be removed; conducting consultations with other physicians; visiting patients at the hospital bed after the operation. Unless doctors find things to do to us, most of them don't get paid.

The result, inevitably, has been an explosion of unnecessary medical services, particularly surgery, often at unreasonably high prices. There are many examples to illustrate this, but none more revealing than the brief history of coronary bypass surgery in the United States.

THE CORONARY BYPASS EPIDEMIC

During coronary bypass surgery, doctors take pieces of vein from a patient's legs and graft them to blocked arteries that supply blood to the heart. The bypass creates a new blood route so the heart muscle does not die for lack of oxygen.

Evidence from a major European study and similar findings of the Veterans Administration and the National Institutes of Health reveal that coronary bypass surgery clearly prolongs life for only about 11 percent of the patients who receive the operation, those whose left main coronary artery is severely obstructed. Bypass surgery may prolong life for 10 to 30 percent more patients— those with obstructions in the three main coronary arteries—but the evidence is inconclusive. Thus, at least 60 percent, and possibly 80 percent, of the 200,000 Americans who submitted to (or in some cases insisted on) coronary bypass surgery in 1984 gained no increase in life span beyond what they would have achieved through medical management of their condition with beta blockers and other modern drugs. Those receiving bypass surgery did subject themselves to special dangers: a 2 percent chance of dying during surgery, a 5 percent risk of a heart attack on the operating table, and a 10 percent chance of a serious complication like stroke, weakening of the heart muscle, or infection. Indeed, for arteries not severely clogged, bypass surgery may increase the rate of blockage. Researchers have found that coronary arteries less than half-blocked were ten times more likely to be completely blocked three years after surgery than those not bypassed.

Although bypass surgery in many cases provides relief from angina, the operation does not cure coronary artery disease. Ten years after surgery, 40 percent of bypass grafts have closed and another 30 percent have narrowed. Repeat surgery is riskier and less effective.

America is in the midst of a coronary bypass epidemic. Americans are four times more likely to have a coronary bypass operation than Western Europeans with the same symptoms, twice as likely as Canadians and Australians. Americans with angina pectoris are ten to twenty times more likely to have a bypass operation than British subjects, at more than ten times the cost. Granted, British physicians have fewer resources available, and the United States has a higher level of heart disease. But these factors are of relatively marginal import. The decisive reason for the vast difference lies in the American fee-for-service payment system. In Europe, Great Britain, and Australia, most doctors get salaries rather than piece rates. So do surgeons and cardiologists working under prepaid plans in the United States, and their patients get coronary bypasses less than half as often as do those who go to fee-for-service doctors.

As Henry Aaron, Senior Fellow at Brookings Institution, and Dr. William Schwartz, professor of medicine at Tufts, put it in their brilliant book, *The Painful Prescription:*

> Most U.S. surgeons are paid on a fee-for-service basis, whereas most British physicians are salaried employees of the NHS [National Health Service]. In close calls the American physician will obviously have a greater incentive to carry out a bypass procedure than his

British counterpart. As one American cardiologist put it: "The entrepreneurial aspect of surgery in this country makes it imperative for surgeons to pursue the recruitment of patients aggressively. There is not only the major income motivation, but also the need to meet all sorts of state standards in terms of the number of cases done per year, solely to justify a cardiac surgical unit's existence.... " [Many states require a hospital to conduct at least 250 heart operations to get a license for a cardiac surgical unit.]

The fees for coronary bypass surgery are plenty high enough to tempt the least knife-happy heart surgeon. Dr. Thomas Preston, chief of cardiology at Seattle's Pacific Medical Center and professor of medicine at the University of Washington, estimates that in 1984 cardiac surgeons' fees for a coronary bypass ran up to $15,000 and averaged around $5,000. At these prices, a surgeon performing 140 bypass operations, about the average, can generate an income of around $700,000, just from those operations. With other fees, Dr. Preston conservatively estimates, total income for these surgeons is at least $750,000, with the specialists most in demand commanding incomes "in the millions."

The total cost of a bypass operation averages about $25,000, with many exceeding $100,000. In 1984 the estimated $5 billion Americans paid for this single procedure accounted for more than 1 percent of our nation's total medical care budget.

By 1984 coronary bypass operations were no longer highly complex; surgical techniques were standardized. The persistently rising cost of the procedure, even after it became routine and surgeons were performing two or three in a day, illustrates the perversity of medical economics. Blue Cross/Blue Shield, private insurers, Medicare, and Medicaid have paid physicians their "usual, customary, and reasonable" fees. Fee reimbursement is measured by what a physician and his colleagues billed in the past, so there's no incentive to lower fees as efficiencies are realized. If anything, under this system the incentive is to raise them, because eventually the historical record of fees billed increases amounts doctors can charge currently and in the future. As long as fees don't exceed the highest range in their market area, the doctors get what they charge. Under a different payment system, the charge of a Canadian surgeon for bypass surgery is about $1,100, roughly one-fifth what U.S. surgeons get.

SHEATHING THE SURGEONS' KNIVES

What happens when the surgeon has no economic incentive to use his knife? The rate of surgery drops sharply and the patients are just as healthy without enduring the risk and pain of the operation. The second-opinion programs of the private insurers and the care of patients who belong to health maintenance organizations demonstrate this.

Under second-opinion programs, whenever a physician recommends surgery, the insurance company pays for another opinion, from an independent physician who has no financial interest in performing the surgery, only a professional interest in the correct medical procedure. I first heard of second-opinion programs when I was Secretary of Health, Education, and Welfare. In our search for ways to reduce health care costs, we discovered that Cornell University Medical College and several local unions had instituted such a program in New York City. According to early returns, surgery was reduced among patients in the program by 10 to 15 percent, with substantial cost savings, because the second opinions frequently concluded that no operation was necessary.

I announced such a program for Medicare, and we ran television commercials to encourage Americans facing one doctor's recommendation for surgery to get the opinion of another, who had no financial incentive to operate. The American Medical Association denounced this effort for fear it would subvert patients' confidence in doctors. But other insurers began to adopt the idea. It is credited with reducing surgery by about 20 percent among patients whose insurance pays for a second opinion. By 1984 three-fourths of the largest commercial group health insurers paid for second opinions to sheath the surgeons' knives when nonemergency surgery was recommended.

There is a vast difference in surgery rates between patients of fee-for-service physicians and patients of health maintenance or-

ganizations, where physicians are paid the same amount regardless
of the services (including surgery) performed. The federal government's employee health plans offer hospitalization under both a
Blue Cross fee-for-service system and an HMO. Consistently, federal employees covered by a Blue Cross fee-for-service plan are
twice as likely to have any given operation, for the same symptoms, as those in the HMO plan. In 1984 a Rand Corporation study
of the Group Health Cooperative of Puget Sound revealed that
this HMO provided full health services for 28 percent less than
fully insured fee-for-service plans for one major reason: HMO
members had 40 percent fewer hospital admissions and hospital
days. Why? Largely because they were subjected to surgical procedures far less often.

WE GET WHAT WE PAY FOR

How doctors are paid can determine how they treat us. Most doctors in the United States are paid a fee for each service performed,
and they like it that way. The fee-for-service medicine men and
women perform more surgery and tests and provide more services
than those who are paid a salary or some flat amount regardless of
the services they give.

Health maintenance organizations do not operate on a fee-for-
service or cost-based reimbursement basis. They commit themselves to provide all the medical care a person or family needs for
a prepaid amount. This eliminates the economic incentive to provide unnecessary services and encourages treatment of illnesses in
the least expensive manner.

The earliest HMOs, then known as prepaid group practices, got
started in 1910, providing at a fixed prearranged price all the
health care needed by employees of some large lumber companies
in Tacoma, Washington. The first HMO characterized as such was
started in 1929 in California, when two doctors contracted with
the Los Angeles Water Department to provide its employees and
their families comprehensive medical services for a single price.
From the beginning, fee-for-service doctors tried to thwart HMOs

by expelling physicians who joined them from state and local medical societies and denying them hospital privileges. Many state legislatures cooperated by enacting "free choice" laws, a euphemism to prohibit formation of HMOs by making it illegal to enter any agreement that limited a patient's right to choose any doctor. Thus, for years in many states, prepaid groups like HMOs, which required the patient to use one of their physician members, were banned because they interfered with the patient's "free choice."

The big breakthrough for HMOs came in 1942, when Henry J. Kaiser formed two, one to provide medical services for Kaiser employees in Portland, Oregon, the other to serve workers in Richmond and Fontana, California. Kaiser was inspired by an HMO set up in 1938 by surgeon Sidney Garfield to provide health care to Kaiser workers building the Grand Coulee Dam. Kaiser and Garfield then brought the concept to other work sites on the West Coast and in 1945 opened Kaiser-Permanente Health Plans to all, first in northern and then in southern California. The concept became more generally accepted in other states as well, notably in Wisconsin and the Minneapolis–St. Paul area of Minnesota, where fully 40 percent of the health care is provided by HMOs.

Still, until the early 1970s, HMOs were not able to shake the label of socialized medicine that fee-for-service doctors and hospital associations had so securely stuck on them. So big business stayed away, especially during the anticommunist fever of the 1950s and 1960s.

It was Richard Nixon's administration that proposed legislation that blessed HMOs. The bill provided that any "federally qualified" HMO (one that met certain health care delivery and financial standards and was approved by the Secretary of HEW) had to be offered to all employees in the geographic area for which it was so qualified. However, a shove from the American Medical Association and its fee-for-service members pushed the Congress and the bureaucracy at the Department of Health, Education, and Welfare to smother the bill in red tape. When I became Secretary in January 1977, I discovered that few HMOs had even sought federal qualification because the average application was a thousand pages long! We cleared out the bureaucracy, simplified the application to less than twenty pages, and campaigned to get existing HMOs qualified and new ones started. Kaiser-Permanente, with its 2.5 million members, qualified and broke the ice for less affluent organizations.

We learned that HMOs needed two other helping hands: capital to start up until they had a large enough patient population to support the doctors, nurses, and equipment they required, and managers who knew how to run efficient business and service delivery operations. I convened a one-day conference on HMOs in 1978 to lure corporate America to take a look, expecting to get a couple of dozen company representatives. More than 600 corporations and unions came, one of the earliest indications that business was beginning to look for less costly ways to provide quality health care to its employees. That was the beginning of the new era for HMOs.

In 1970 less than fifteen states had HMOs. By 1984 forty-one states and the District of Columbia had such organizations. In 1970 HMOs could claim barely 3 million members. By 1984 all but one of the nation's thirty-eight major metropolitan areas had at least one HMO, and almost 17 million Americans were members. The biggest jump came in 1984, as enrollments increased by more than 22 percent and corporations energetically promoted prepaid plans. Dr. Paul Ellwood, head of a health research firm and an early proponent of prepaid group practice, believes that more than 50 million Americans will belong to HMOs by 1993. For-profit HMOs are popping up across America, with several making public stock offerings in 1984 and 1985 at dizzying price-to-earnings ratios.

The success of HMOs in holding down costs has prompted business not only to use them, but also to spur other competition with fee-for-service doctors by financing preferred providers. Such providers contract directly with a corporation or insurance company to furnish medical services at a prearranged, usually discounted, cost, either for an individual or family, or for specific services. The number of Americans getting health care through preferred providers soared from 1.3 million to 5.8 million in the first half of 1985, a more than fourfold increase.

THE FREEDOM-OF-CHOICE MYTH

Fee-for-service doctors intone as sacred chant "freedom of choice," the right of patients to choose any doctor they want, to be bankrolled by third-party payers. But that choice is hardly real. It may provide some psychic succor, but as Willis Goldbeck, president of the Washington Business Group on Health, points out, that's about all it offers.

Most patients choose their family doctor. Beyond that, the family doctor chooses all the specialists and surgeons, who in turn select the anesthesiologists, radiologists, pathologists, hospitals, and nurses. But the selection of a family doctor can hardly be considered a well-informed free choice.

As intelligent choice requires information, and the fee-for-service doctors take every step possible to deny us that information. If the customer has no information about quality or price, how can he or she make a free choice among alternatives? But patients in the United States have no information about individual doctor's hospitalization and surgery practices; morbidity and mortality rates for different diseases; methods of treatment; charges for medical tests, diagnosis, and procedures; use of drugs or surgery for particular diagnoses, as compared with the practice of other doctors. We do not even know which doctors perform a sufficient number of open-heart or stomach cancer operations to get the optimal results, or what the costs and medical procedures are at the hospitals where they do their surgery.

There's nothing special about medical suppliers, such as doctors and hospitals, that gives them the right to deny us the kind of information we would demand from any other seller. They can provide such information in ways that protect patient privacy. Without it, freedom of choice is a game of blind man's bluff, with patients blindfolded, spun around a few times, and then sent in a general direction and told to pin the Blue Cross/Blue Shield card on the doctor.

In April of 1985, the Department of Health and Human Services issued a regulation requiring public access to statistics showing how well hospitals treat various illnesses. The information is to be made available by peer review organizations created by Congress to monitor hospitals' services to Medicare patients. The information, including admission rates, lengths of stay, prevalence of hospital-acquired infections, and death rates for different departments and illnesses, should help consumers to evaluate hospital performance. However, the regulation does not apply to doctors, and none will be identified by name.

THE DENTISTS

In some ways, the dental industry represents a doctor's nightmare come true. The fact that too many dentists compete to fix fewer unhealthy teeth has held their income to about the level of general inflation, set off price competition, and sparked new delivery systems.

Overall, the business of dentistry has been expanding steadily, from $2.8 billion in 1965 to $25 billion in 1984, and is expected to reach some $40 billion by 1990. But since 1972, the number of dentists has increased twice as fast as the general population has. In 1972 there was one dentist for every 2,000 Americans; in 1984 there was one for about every 1,700. This rise was prompted in part by the same 1965 Health Professions Educational Assistance legislation that set off the increase in the number of doctors.

Americans paid 400 million visits to almost 140,000 dentists' offices in 1984, about 1.7 visits per person. Half our population do not see a dentist during a year, while only a quarter go a year without seeing a doctor. At an average of 5.7 visits per capita, doctors get far more repeat business. Dentists, with net income averaging $60,000, earn only about half of what the average doctor makes.

While the overall health of Americans has shown improvement over the past two decades, dental health has made enormous strides, thanks largely to widespread fluoridation of the water supply. Cavities are becoming extinct: tooth decay has dropped 50 percent since the 1960s; one of three college-age Americans has never had a cavity; and new antiplaque discoveries augur another major prevention tool to further reduce the need for dental services.

Dentists have not been able to get securely hitched to the third-party, usual, customary, and reasonable fee payment system, and it shows. Unlike doctors, 70 percent of whose income is paid by government or private insurers, America's 140,000 dentists get only a third of their income from third parties.

Dental insurance plans do cover an increasing number of people, up from 17 million in 1972 to about 100 million in 1984. In 1972 patients directly paid 90 percent of their dental bills; in 1984 patients paid about two-thirds of their bills. By 1990 the patient share is projected to drop to about 62 percent. The demand for dental services, which once fluctuated with the business cycle, continued to rise during the 1981–1982 recession, indicating that the growth of third-party coverage for dental services is starting to create some of the same utilization ripples it has for doctors.

But competition among dentists and the lessons of runaway physician costs have led corporate employers, who set the pace, to look to HMO-type dental plans to control costs. Seven to 10 percent of Americans with dental insurance are enrolled in a plan offering to provide all dental services for a fixed predetermined fee. Although, like doctors, many dentists have resisted prepayment plans, the growing supply of dentists and the push of corporate America for such plans appears to guarantee their acceptance.

ARE DOCTORS GOOD GUYS OR BAD GUYS?

It's not that doctors wear black hats and the rest of us wear white ones. The overwhelming majority of physicians, like other health professionals, take their responsibilities seriously. They do all they know how to do for those who seek their help. The training is long, often tedious, persistently arduous. Many, particularly those in pediatrics, family practice, and other primary care roles, spend long hours on the job and are often consulted at all hours of the night. Specialists at topflight medical centers like Memorial Sloan-Kettering start before dawn and serve patients long into the night. Many physicians devote their lives to public service and the poor, at the National Institutes of Health, in public hospitals and clinics, at the Defense Department, and in the Public Health Service.

On average, doctors report a work week of fifty-seven hours, fifty-one of which are devoted to patient care. They know that their actions can drastically, sometimes irrevocably, change the quality of life for a patient, even determine whether an individual will live or die. That's a big part of the reason why they don't want to overlook any test or treatment that might benefit their patients.

The winds of change bedevil the medical profession. The rapid growth of medical knowledge, new technology, including computers that are revolutionizing the way doctors diagnose and decide how to treat patients, specialization, urbanization, cultural revolution, drugs, the increasing oversupply of doctors, the pressure to curtail costs and cut waste, and a host of other forces over which physicians can exercise little control and from which they find it increasingly difficult to get shelter have turned the doctor with the little black bag and stethoscope into an anachronism, a figure from a Norman Rockwell *Saturday Evening Post* cover whose prototype even Grandpa has difficulty remembering.

In 1984 just under half of all active physicians remained in fee-for-service solo operations, a far cry from 1935, when 95 percent were going it alone. Twenty-five percent were in fee-for-service group practices, 13 percent in HMOs, and the rest were associated with preferred provider organizations and/or freestanding emergency centers.

For years, physicians have regulated themselves and controlled the health care system in which they worked and made money. They not only set the course of treatment for all patients but played the decisive role in every phase of the organization and management of health care. Doctors alone determined the scope and content of education in medical schools and on-the-job training in hospitals. Doctors decided who should practice medicine and who should not. They also circumscribed the scope of practice of all other health professionals, by the simple but powerful tool of defining just what the practice of medicine is and getting state legislators to make that practice their exclusive prerogative. For decades, they controlled and allocated most hospital resources.

But the medical times, they are a-changing. Medical schools are beginning to respond to the need for doctors trained in health promotion and disease prevention. In the fall of 1985, Harvard

Medical School dean Daniel Tosteson introduced a New Pathway curriculum. This education program, for twenty-four of the seventy-two first-year students, de-emphasizes large lectures, avoids information overload, and encourages closer student contact with faculty and patients. Students start by doing a health risk assessment of themselves and calculating the effects that various risk factors will have on their own life spans. Throughout the four-year curriculum, these students will work continually with some patients and families and provide health-promotion services at the Harvard Community Health Plan, an HMO associated with the medical school. Dr. Tosteson's goal is to integrate health promotion with every facet of medical education. He hopes the entire student body will be taking the New Pathway curriculum by 1990.

The third-party reimbursement system that doctors helped shape to assure payment of whatever usual, customary, and reasonable fees they billed is coming back to bite the hands it filled with money. Because corporations and governments now pay most bills, the physicians are losing their singularly potent economic leverage: the fact that individual patients, from whom most of the money once came, were unable to organize effectively as consumers. In the 1980s only pediatricians receive more than half their income directly from patients. On average, doctors receive 44 percent of their income from commercial insurers and Blue Shield (most of which ultimately comes from large corporations and unions), 28 percent from Medicare and Medicaid, and 28 percent from patients. These large institutional third parties who pick up some 70 percent of the bills are increasingly resistant to paying for wasteful practices and unnecessary surgery. They have concluded that medicine is too important and expensive to leave to the doctors, just as war is too important to leave to the generals.

The large corporate buyers and insurers of health care have reached this conclusion not because they believe doctors are villains. Rather, they have finally recognized that doctors, like the rest of us, will act according to the economic and professional incentives they face. Doctors are trained to treat sick people, not to prevent disease or promote healthy life-styles. The economic system in which they work pays them for providing medical services; for most doctors, the more services they provide, the more money they make. The more specialized they are, the higher the fees they can charge and the more prestige they have in their profession and their communities.

Doctors are giving patients what they want. The spurt in cesarean deliveries is far more pronounced in suburbia and affluent sections of cities. In upper-class and upper-middle-class America, such deliveries have become fashionable, culturally as well as medically. Many family physicians dispense sleeping pills and Valium to adult patients the way indulgent parents give gumdrops to their children, because those patients want instant relief from the stress of modern life. In areas where doctors should say no, every economic and professional incentive, right down to keeping the well-insured patient as a customer, encourages them to say yes.

So, the doctor. The medicine men and women of America.

Are they important?

You bet. It's hard to change the health care system without them—as most of us who've tried have learned.

We're coming to appreciate that, like most Americans, doctors will respond to financial incentives far more readily than they will accept regulation. We can change the economic bait for our physicians. In a time shorter than most Americans think possible, that will change the way doctors practice medicine.

Dr. James Sammons, the shrewd, pragmatic, committed executive vice-president of the American Medical Association, senses this. That's why he calls these years "the toughest times for doctors" in the history of America. He's right. And they're likely to get tougher.

Chapter 6

THE TEMPLES OF
THE MEDICINE MEN

If doctors are the high priests of medicine, hospitals are their temples.

Hospitals are the heavy industry of the health care economy. Intensively capitalized with their elaborate buildings and sophisticated equipment, they took 40 percent of the money we spent on health care in 1984. The best of them attract the best and the brightest—and the most richly rewarded—of the medical profession. They are the most expensive component of the health care complex.

It wasn't always so.

At the midpoint of the nineteenth century, people went to hospitals to die, or because they had no one to care for them at home. At best, hospital care was palliative. It was rarely curative. At worst, and quite frequently, it was deadly.

By the midpoint of the twentieth century, hospitals had been transformed. Today, they are gleaming temples of hope, staffed by professionals as highly trained and accomplished as any society produces, stocked with some of the highest of high-tech equipment.

Of the 6,900 hospitals in the United States, about 5,800 are community hospitals.* Of these community hospitals, about 1,700

* Of the remaining 1,100, 580 are psychiatric hospitals, 400 are run by the Department of Defense, the Veterans Administration, the National Institutes of Health, and other government agencies; and 120 are dedicated to special treatment of tuberculosis and respiratory and other diseases.

(with 20 percent of the beds) are public hospitals owned and operated mostly by cities and counties, but also by states, at a cost approaching $20 billion in 1984. About 3,300 are nonprofit, including about 1,000 affiliated with religious groups, mostly Catholic. Some 800 are operated for a profit.

The 5,800 community hospitals provide short-term care, usually for less than thirty days. They are the focal point for the delivery of high-tech, high-cost health care to nearly 25 million people, who account for 36 million admissions each year. Millions more make some 300 million outpatient visits annually. In 1984, at these hospitals surgeons performed 20 million operations, and 3.5 million children were born.

The single most common reason for hospitalization is childbirth, which represents about 10 percent of all admissions. Heart diseases lead the list of ailments for which people are hospitalized, responsible for about 8 percent; cancer is responsible for 5 percent of all admissions; bone fractures, cerebrovascular disease, and pneumonia each account for 2 to 3 percent.

Citizens aged sixty-five and older account for almost one-third of the hospital admissions each year, although they make up only about 12 percent of the population. They have the longest average length of stay in the hospital. About 18 percent of their admissions are related to heart diseases, 9 percent to cancer, 6 percent to cerebrovascular diseases, and 3 percent to pneumonia. The 5 percent of patients with catastrophic, high-cost illnesses, most of them elderly, account for 30 percent of total hospital charges.

For men fifteen to forty-four years old, alcohol dependence is the second-highest reason for admission listed on hospital records; for men forty-five to sixty-four, it is the fourth highest. But many, perhaps even most, admissions actually due to alcohol abuse, ranging from cirrhosis of the liver to accidents, are not so attributed.

To do their work, hospitals employ some 4.3 million Americans, an annual payroll of more than $60 billion. The ratio of staff to patient in American hospitals has been approaching four to one. There's nothing like our hospital staffing in the rest of the world, even in countries with health care systems as advanced as ours. In West Germany, where doctors are counted as staff, the ratio is one to one; in Great Britain, the Netherlands, and Belgium, two to one.

IN THE GOOD OLD COST-PLUS DAYS

While hospitals have steadily eaten up 40 percent of the total health care bill, they have taken a persistently increasing share of our personal health care bill: from 35 percent in 1950 to 47 percent in 1984. By 1990 hospitals could take half of all the money Americans spend on personal health care.

Over the ten years preceding 1984, total hospital charges have increased at an average annual rate of nearly 15 percent, outpacing all other segments of the health care industry along the inflation road. From 1965 to 1984, the cost of care has increased ten times, from an average of $41 for each hospital day to $432; it is projected to reach $800 per day by 1990. The price of an average stay, now almost $3,000, could easily top $5,000 in 1990.

Much of this stunning increase is attributable to the third-party, cost-based reimbursement system and the fact that hospitals have regarded doctors, not patients, as their customers.

Hospital administrators look to doctors for the patients to fill their beds, and doctors, as the perceived customers of hospitals, control most of what goes on there. Doctors tend to view hospitals as free workshops; their incentive has been to hospitalize patients whenever medically desirable, whether or not medically necessary. The patients, whose insurers are paying most of the bills, are the doctors' clients, not the hospitals'. Patients have little capacity to assess the cost-effectiveness of their care, and when well insured, they have no incentive to do so.

The cost-based, third-party system of payment used with few exceptions until 1984, insulated hospital administrators from any need to worry about costs, whether for nurses and other staff, expensive equipment, linens, heat, or empty space. There was no incentive to seek competitive bids from qualified suppliers. There was little reason to operate efficiently, plan ahead, or buy prudently. Equipment could be depreciated gradually, or written off as soon as newer models came on the market. It all went into the costs for which hospitals were reimbursed.

Indeed, there was the perverse incentive to use the equipment to run tests. The more tests, the more revenue for the hospital. And to admit patients. The more patients, the more revenue for the hospital. And to keep patients in the hospital. The more days, the more costs to be reimbursed.

Our health insurance system has been so tilted toward hospital reimbursement that it has paid physicians more for services rendered in hospitals than for those performed in their offices. It has been the catastrophic event we feared most and against which we insured—the heart attack or serious accident. Eventually, this tilt encouraged doctors to treat patients in hospitals: after all, patients wouldn't have to pay out-of-pocket as much as they would for outpatient care, which was far less comprehensively insured, and the doctor got higher fees. Even after accounting for differences in the complexity of treatment, physicians get four to five times more for an hour of surgery conducted in hospitals than for taking an hour in their offices to analyze a case and persuade a patient to adopt healthier habits. Medicare has paid 20 to 30 percent more for nonsurgical services provided in a hospital. When these higher rates of reimbursement are combined with the time savings from seeing patients on hospital rounds, doctors can boost their hourly earnings by as much as 100 percent by working in the hospital.

More than 26 percent of American doctors have financial arrangements with hospitals that encourage them to admit patients and test them there. These relationships, especially for traditionally hospital-based specialties like pathology and radiology, can be very lucrative. Although, under pressure from Medicare, the practice seems to be declining, many doctors have been paid a percentage of the gross fees generated by their departments, whether or not they personally perform each procedure. Hospital-based physicians with percentages of the gross often earn twice as much as salaried doctors in the same specialties.

MEDICAL FEATHERBEDDING

The existence of such incentives explains in large measure why there has been so much medical featherbedding—why we are so frequently stuck with needles and X-rayed, so endlessly tested and sampled once we walk through the doors of a hospital. These ancillary services, as hospital administrators call them, typically account for 40 to 50 percent of those whopping hospital bills most patients never read.

Buried in a 1983 report of the President's Commission for the Study of Ethical Problems in Medical and Biological and Behavioral Research, and scattered throughout other studies, are these revelations of medical featherbedding:

- Some 20 percent of the days patients spend in hospitals are unnecessary.
- Although automation of laboratory analyses has lowered the cost of individual tests, cost-based reimbursement encourages hospitals to increase the number of tests done rather than reduce patients' hospital bills.
- Extra hospital tests increase the likelihood of "false positive" results, which then lead to further testing and clinical evaluation, and hence more unnecessary costs.
- A study by doctors at the University of California–San Francisco concluded that eliminating unnecessary tests before surgery could save $1 billion a year.
- Many patients now admitted to hospital intensive care units don't need anything like the level of services such units provide. Since costs in these units are up to five times those in regular hospital rooms, a more careful selection of patients could save billions and would spare many patients the isolation and stress that such units create.
- At least 35 percent of the special respiratory care treatments and tests for breathing and oxygen, now given to one of every four hospitalized patients and often involving sophisticated machinery, are unnecessary. The savings would be about $1.5 billion if we eliminated such unneeded care.
- A group of specialists convened by the National Institutes of Health in 1984 found that blood plasma transfusions are used un-

necessarily 90 percent of the time, an enormous waste and risk of transmitting disease.

THE MEDICAL ARMS RACE

The fat years of cost and cost-plus reimbursement provided a rich market for every diagnostic and therapeutic weapon American manufacturers could invent, and relieved manufacturers of any concerns about the relationship between costs and benefits. As long as they sold their inventions to hospitals, the price was irrelevant. The hospitals wanted to keep up with the Joneses. So one CAT (computerized axial tomography) scanner led to another; one intensive care unit or cardiology department to another. Atlanta has more CAT scanners than all of Connecticut; southern California more than are needed west of the Mississippi.

The hospitals, indeed, had powerful motivation to buy the latest, the best, the gold-plated version of every medical weapon. They wanted the best doctors, who could guarantee them patients. To get them, hospitals bought every medical gadget the doctors asked for. Many physicians became like caricatures of Latin American and Middle Eastern generals who were offered ever more sophisticated and expensive weaponry by the United States and Russia to lure them to the American or Soviet side. Like the generals, the physicians didn't care about cost; they weren't paying for the machinery. Nor did the hospital, because it got its money back, whatever it paid. With Medicare and Medicaid, the U.S. government bankrolled the purchase of diagnostic and therapeutic weapons, as hospitals vied with each other for the latest stuff. We created a medical arms race, as intensely competitive as any military arms race.

It was inevitable that the medical arms race would escalate to the world of helicopters. By 1984 more than a hundred hospitals had their own choppers. Hospitals buy helicopters at a cost of $1 million to $2 million apiece, or lease them from companies that provide helicopter services for hospitals. Hermann Hospital in Houston, Texas, has five choppers that fly 3,200 missions per year at an annual operating cost exceeding $2 million. The hospital bills patients up to $2,000 a ride, a charge usually covered by insurance. We learned in the Vietnam War that prompt treatment can be of the essence in life-threatening situations, such as severe burn cases. But that does not require neighboring hospitals each to have its own helicopter unit. Too often those units are used more for glamour and prestige than to save lives. In September 1984, the Washington, D.C., Hospital Center used two helicopters to fly five Maryland state legislators to a luncheon and tour of its facilities. The purpose? To lobby for rules to increase the number of Maryland patients flown to its shock-trauma center!

Helicopters neatly fit the military analogy, but they are not the costliest new medical weapons. The top spots belong to new diagnostic inventions. Among the latest and most expensive are the NMRs—the nuclear magnetic resonance scanners. In late 1984 the industry dropped "nuclear" from the scanner's name to avoid the potentially negative association with nuclear war, waste, and plants, and began calling them MRs. These machines display a three-dimensional cross section of the part of the body they view. The MR produces images of soft tissue, a major advance in detecting head and neck injuries, abscesses, and tumors. We are just beginning to realize the benefits of this new technology—including its potential to reduce uncertainty and unnecessary surgery—but its costs are already apparent. The average cost for a hospital to purchase and install an MR is over $2 million. It takes at least $4 million to get top-of-the-line models. Everybody wants one.

By 1984 more than 150 MRs were in place and twenty of the top thirty insurance companies were paying $500 to $1,400 a scan. A hospital must scan six to twelve patients daily to break even on their investment within the usual five-to-seven-year depreciation period. Many, however, were performing four or fewer scans per day in 1984.

The top-dollar kid on the block of diagnostic scanners gives some sense of how far we can go to spend money in this area. PETs—positive emission tomographers—are coming. By the end of 1984, more than six medical centers had them and a number of others were waiting in line. They are remarkable medical detectives that reveal all sorts of information about chemical activity,

show what parts of the brain you use when you move an arm or leg
or think, and diagnose certain kinds of heart and brain disease and
cancer. But PETs have expensive taste. They need to be near a cyclotron. The combined cost of the PET and the cyclotron ap-
proaches $5 million; cyclotrons alone cost at least $1,000 per hour
to run. PETs can do much diagnostic good, but a PET scan could
also cost $7,000 to $10,000 to locate an irreversible cancer or to
detect that loss of memory was due to an incurable disease.

MRs and PETs are the latest entries in the medical arms race of
high-tech diagnostic procedures. These scanners augment a huge
arsenal of ultrasound and X-ray devices. The very existence of
such technology in a cost-based, fully insured payment system,
with doctors rightly worried about malpractice lawsuits, has encouraged promiscuous use. Hospitals do 200 million X-rays, CAT
scans, and other diagnostic scans each year, at a cost of $7 billion.
These procedures account for 3 to 5 percent of total hospital expenditures, and their use has been growing at an 8 percent annual
rate.

It's not just the cost of new diagnostic devices that kicks up the
nation's health bill. Too frequently, these machines do not replace
old procedures they do more effectively; they simply augment
them. This is particularly true in the diagnosis and treatment of
women. Blue Cross investigations reveal that women often receive
a battery of tests to evaluate breast disease—mammography, ultrasound, thermography, diaphanography, and more—where one
correctly chosen procedure would suffice.

The use of high-technology imaging became so excessive in
1984 that Blue Cross/Blue Shield issued guidelines, stopping payments for duplicative diagnostic procedures and for the inexcus-
ably wasteful use of expensive CAT scans to diagnose complaints
such as simple headaches. The General Accounting Office, an investigative arm of the Congress, also found that about 9 percent of
Medicare's diagnostic radiology charges were for unnecessary
procedures.

Advanced diagnostic techniques are valuable; they save lives
and can help direct the doctor more surely to appropriate treatment. These inventions are part of what makes ours the finest
medical system in the world. Used efficiently, they can improve

the quality of care and at the same time reduce costs by directing doctors away from unnecessary medical procedures. But their overuse wastes money. Britain performs roughly one-half the number of X-ray examinations per capita, using one-quarter the film at one-seventh of the cost.

The same sort of profligacy that abounds in the diagnosis of hospital patients pops up repeatedly in their care. Intensive care units (ICUs) and coronary care units (CCUs) are the sophisticated nuclear aircraft carriers of American hospitals. Nowhere has the medical arms race escalated so rapidly, so wastefully, and at such high cost.

Hospitals have been adding intensive care beds at an average rate of more than 2,500 a year since 1958. There are about 70,000 hospital beds in intensive and coronary care units. This 7 percent of all beds accounts for 20 percent of all hospital charges.

Intensive and coronary care units provide critical care to the dangerously ill. Patients admitted to intensive care units receive up to thirty-five active life-support therapies, and more nursing care than is normally available. Patients suffering from heart attacks, other serious coronary conditions, severe asthma, gastrointestinal bleeding, and acute liver and kidney failure belong in these units at critical moments. But many stable patients are admitted routinely after major surgery to avoid any malpractice claims, and a substantial number of patients admitted are elderly, in chronically poor health, with little chance for short-term survival. Although proportions vary from hospital to hospital, nationally about 40 percent of patients admitted to intensive care units have had complicated surgery or require close monitoring for other reasons. The other 60 percent tend to be very sick, in acute and terminal phases of chronic diseases like kidney failure or cirrhosis. The average length of stay in such units is about 3.5 days; patients admitted for monitoring average about 2 days, while those with chronic diseases may remain for weeks.

Intensive care units offer a continuous electrocardiogram for each patient and most patients are so monitored. Pacemakers, defibrillators (machines that deliver electrical impulses to the heart), ventilators (machines that maintain breathing), kidney dialysis machines, and other life-support equipment are readily available, as is X-ray and other diagnostic equipment. Many units have their own laboratories. Closed-circuit television and computer monitoring provide so much data on patient condition that doctors and nurses often suffer from information overload.

Intensive care units use three times the number of nursing hours per patient-day as general medical and surgical wards and employ far more doctors, laboratory technicians, and computer and clerical personnel.

These units have saved lives that would otherwise have been lost. But once again, the cost-based, third-party reimbursement system has encouraged unnecessary use at exorbitant cost. In 1983 George Washington University doctors investigated the use of intensive care units. They discovered widespread unnecessary use of intensive care therapy in hospitals. They found that reducing the number of patients admitted—including those too sick or not sick enough to benefit from such expensive care—would cut money spent for such units by 15 percent. In terms of the nation's 1984 hospital bill, proper use of these units would have saved $2.1 billion.

There is room for savings even when patients are properly admitted to intensive care units. With the cost-based, third-party reimbursement system, the tendency has been to give all intensive care patients every service and monitor available. The same George Washington University study found that reducing the intensity of care in "extravagant" hospitals would save an additional $1.4 billion, with no adverse impact on medical outcomes. Unnecessary use of pulmonary-artery catheters provides a good example. These devices measure differences in blood pressure between the left and right sides of the heart. Two million are used each year at a direct cost approaching $2 billion, with another $1 billion for increased nursing and complications the device itself causes. Depending on the hospital involved, these catheters are not needed in 10 to 33 percent of the cases in which they're used. The fact that some hospitals use these devices two to three times more often than others to treat the same symptoms and with no difference in therapeutic results signals great waste and the potential for big savings.

The urgency of confronting the profligacy of American hospital care is accentuated by the speed with which our scientific gurus produce new technology. The Congressional Office of Technology Assessment found that 30 percent of the more than doubling of Medicare's costs from 1977 to 1982 was due to new technology and drugs. Medical scholar and clinician Dr. William Schwartz believes that "the growth of technology is faster than at any time in . . . 25 years." If any proof is needed that the financial problem is here to stay—along with a baffling grid of human and moral issues—just consider the fact that the main limit on the number of transplants is now lack of available organs.

Heart transplants cost at least $100,000, and many cost several times that amount. About 175 were performed in 1984. The total would jump to at least 10,000 each year if sufficient hearts were available.

Liver transplants cost an average of $135,000 each. First-year rehabilitation costs can raise this to $300,000. About 160 were performed in 1984. The number would nudge 5,000 each year if enough organs were available.

Kidney transplants cost up to $40,000. Some 6,000 were performed in 1984. With more organs, the total number would more than double.

Pancreas transplants cost up to $50,000. Two hundred were performed in 1984. Many surgeons believe there would be 10,000 candidates a year if they had the organs.

Future technology will permit hospitals to offer everything from artificial hearts to ear and eye implants for the deaf and the blind, to replacing severed limbs. These medical miracles offer hope for a better life to thousands of human beings, and for the patients served they will be well worth the expense. They can come at such towering cost that it will press our society, in the words of President Derek Bok of Harvard, to face "the problem of deciding what price to put upon a human life."

It won't be easy to slow or even rationalize the medical arms race. I know that not only from my hard public knocks as Secretary of Health, Education, and Welfare, but in my private life as well.

In the spring of 1984 David Axelrod, New York State's health commissioner, denied Memorial Sloan-Kettering in Manhattan the right to buy an expensive MR scanner because New York Hospital, just across the street, already had one. Within forty-eight hours, my wife, Hilary, a trustee of the hospital, received a frantic letter from Dr. Paul Marks, Sloan-Kettering's administrator. What did Dr. Marks suggest? Write to New York State Governor Mario Cuomo, of course—the suggestion he made to each member of Memorial's influential, blue-chip board of trustees. My wife immediately sent this handwritten letter:

> Dear Governor Cuomo:
> I sit on the Board of Memorial Sloan-Kettering Cancer Center and am deeply disturbed that the center was not selected to participate in the N.M.R. demonstration project. We are the major cancer center of the world. Memorial is one of the treasures of New York State, and its work has saved thousands of lives.
> The State should judge the hospital's need for complex, expensive equipment in the context of Memorial Sloan-Kettering as a unique research center, not just another hospital.
> I urge you to review the decision made by Dr. David Axelrod, Commissioner of New York State's Department of Health, and reverse it.
>
> Sincerely yours,
>
> Hilary Paley Califano

Weeks later, New York State permitted Sloan-Kettering to have its MR scanner, saving face by insisting that the purchase be made without borrowing. The state claimed that eliminating the expense of borrowing cut the cost of a single MR scan from $641 to $325 (a claim that ignores the fungibility of money).

THE EMERGENCY ROOM

Have you ever rushed your child to a hospital emergency room with a cut hand, split lip, or broken arm? Most of us with children have. But how many of us have looked at the bill?

These are cases where emergency care is needed—although

even in the cited examples, the cost of care is high. Far more troubling is the fact that 50 percent of the patients treated in emergency rooms don't need such expensive care. The President's Commission for the Study of Ethical Problems found that "about half the patients treated in hospital emergency rooms are not urgently in need of care; many could receive better care at lower cost in a setting expressly designed for routine ambulatory care."

How much could be saved? One survey found that treatment of bronchitis or upper respiratory infection cost $136 at a hospital emergency room, compared with $34 at a freestanding center; a simple arm fracture cost $157 to treat in an emergency room, $71 in a freestanding center; influenza with fever, $159 vs. $30; laceration of arm, $133 vs. $75; corneal abrasion, $97 vs. $40.

TOO MANY ADMISSIONS

The experience of companies like Chrysler and studies sponsored by the Department of Health and Human Services and the General Accounting Office indicate that 20 to 25 percent of all hospital admissions never should have taken place. These studies mean that in 1984 Americans were committed to hospitals six million times when they never should have gone.

Aside from the unnecessary emotional trauma and physical pain and risk to which millions of individuals were subjected, the cost of unnecessary hospital admissions in 1984 is estimated at $30 billion.

TOO MUCH TIME

Those properly admitted to hospitals have been kept there too long. U.S. Health Care Financing Administration studies discovered that one out of every five days properly admitted Medicare and Medicaid patients spend in hospitals are unnecessary.

These unnecessary days have come either at the beginning of the hospital stay, when, for example, patients have been admitted on a Friday or Saturday even though no one will be around to do anything until Monday (a revenue-raising gimmick many hospitals have used), or at the end of the stay, when patients are kept longer than necessary for their treatment. Sunrise Hospital in Las Vegas, Nevada, held a lottery for a cruise for two in the Caribbean for patients who checked in on weekends (which gave the hospital one or two days of full charges with few services to provide). In eighteen months, largely because of weekend check-ins, admissions jumped by 60 percent.

Patients kept too long often want to be there. For instance, women who have just given birth, or older people recovering from surgery, frequently want to "rest up" for an extra day or two (or more) before returning home to other children or to a lonely life. Doctors tend to accede to these requests when they're not paying the bills; fully insured patients tend to make them when they don't think they are either.

TOO MANY BEDS

With occupancy rates of about 75 percent in 1982, former U.S. Surgeon General Julius Richmond concluded that we had 150,000 too many hospital beds in America. By 1984 occupancy rates had dropped to almost 66 percent, leaving us with at least another 50,000 excess beds. Eliminating those 200,000 excess beds, each costing about $30,000 per year, could save us about $6 billion. Moreover, a major factor in hospital admissions has been the number of available beds: the more beds, the more admissions.

Although the number of community hospitals has remained constant since 1972, the number of beds in those hospitals has gone up by more than 100,000. In 1984 America had 4.2 community hospital beds for every 1,000 citizens (probably more, since hospitals take beds out of use in times of low demand and reactivate them when demand picks up). The excess is not evenly distributed; some cities, like St. Louis, have 5.6 beds per 1,000 or more. In New York City, 25 percent of the hospital beds are estimated to be unnecessary. A Maryland state-sponsored study in

1985 found that one-third of the state's 15,000 general hospital beds were unnecessary and recommended closing fourteen hospitals and eliminating hundreds of beds in others.

Willis Goldbeck, president of the Washington Business Group on Health, predicts that lots of hospitals with 50 to 60 percent occupancy rates will close down. If Goldbeck and others who make the same prognosis are correct, we will realize the savings from a more intelligent use of medical resources rather than simply spread the cost over fewer beds.

While I was HEW Secretary in the late 1970s, the outside estimate of the maximum number of beds needed was 4 per 1,000; the number in a reasonably efficient system is much lower. As HMO care, with its lower hospitalization rates, covers more people, and as government and business push to eliminate unnecessary hospitalization, far fewer beds will be required.

But closing hospitals is hard labor. Even converting them to other uses, such as long-term care, requires a cumbersome bureaucratic process in several states. Attempts to close hospitals meet with fierce community resistance—even when the community is told—as the citizens of Seneca Falls, New York, were in 1962 before their hospital was built—that occupancy rates at existing hospitals are low. Everyone admits we have too many hospital beds in America—they're just all in someone else's town, city, or neighborhood.

The desirability of reducing the number of hospital beds and consolidating facilities is not limited to cost savings. Concentration of surgical procedures in fewer hospitals will mean better medical care. Patients are more likely to die in hospitals with low occupancy rates, where fewer operations are performed. A study of 266,944 patients at 1,244 hospitals undertaken by the U.S. Department of Health and Human Services revealed that patients undergoing surgery had a 13 percent greater chance of dying if the surgery was performed at hospitals that did relatively fewer operations. The operations reviewed were common ones: surgery involving the gall bladder, ulcers, the large bowel, and the intra-abdominal artery; arthoplasty of the hip; two types of hip fractures; and two types of lower-limb amputations. Projected nationally, the study suggests that in 1984, 3,000 to 4,000 patients died unnecessarily—just because their operations were performed at hospitals with too little surgical experience. This extensive study confirmed earlier smaller-scale investigations. So, for the health and indeed the lives of our people, as well as to lower costs, it is critical to close unnecessary beds.

BIZARRE BUYING, BILLING, AND BOOKKEEPING

Hospitals have been ineffective in holding down the prices of mundane goods and services they buy. In a cost-reimbursement system, there have been few incentives to haggle over the price of Band-Aids, pacemakers, cleaning fluid, Kleenex, linens, and other sundries. Yet prudent purchasing can produce results, even on small items. In 1984, Northwestern Memorial Hospital in Chicago solicited competing bids from suppliers of surgical gloves. The hospital lowered its cost by more than 10 percent, from 37 to 33 cents a pair, for savings of $11,240, on the more than 280,000 gloves it uses each year.

Noncompetitive billing practices are exposed in hospital charges like these: a 69-cent charge for a single Tylenol pill; a $1.70 charge for one digoxin tablet, a heart stimulant that sells in pharmacies for about 7 cents; charges for electrocardiograms ranging from $67.75 to $155 (a Washington, D.C., commercial laboratory bills $42); charges for an electrolyte panel, a blood test for certain chemicals, ranging from $40.12 to $101 (the same test costs $8.75 at a commercial laboratory); charges by a Florida hospital of $1 each for cotton balls, which retail at 350 for 79 cents; a hospital charge to a sixty-seven-year-old woman for a pregnancy test before routine surgery (Medicare paid it after the hospital rejected her argument that it was ridiculous); a $75 charge for "traction" during hospital treatment for bunions (the "traction" turned out to be the patient's use of a small, baby-size pillow).

The lack of businesslike techniques is also evident in error rates in hospital billings that result in overcharges of 5 to 15 percent of a typical bill. Equifax Services, Incorporated, which specializes in auditing large hospital bills for insurance companies, uncovered overcharges in more than 97 percent of such bills it examined in

1984. Other studies reveal the average hospital bill has $600 in overcharges, owing mainly to misplaced zeros and full-term charges for drugs or services discontinued during recuperation. One patient at a Virginia hospital received one unit of albumin, but his insurance company was charged for 111 units at $56 per unit. In California, a man who refused a hospital's ambulance service and drove his wife to the hospital found that his insurance company was billed $600 for the ambulance ride that never occurred. Another hospital charged $35 to circumcise a newborn girl. By 1984 there were several dozen companies specializing in auditing hospital bills. They claim a saving of $3 for every $1 spent on their services.

BIG BUSINESS GOES TO THE HOSPITAL

The biggest growth in the health industry has been in the for-profit area. In 1983, 141 medical product and service companies went public, compared with 31 in 1982. This growth mirrors what's happening in health care generally. In 1984 there were approximately 100 publicly held health care companies with stock worth $22 billion.

The fastest-growing hospitals have been those run for a profit. There are about 1,100 for-profit community and special-purpose hospitals. For-profit community hospitals grew from 775 with 70,000 beds in 1974 to 816 with 125,000 beds in 1984. Over this same period, the total number of community hospitals and hospital beds dropped slightly. For-profit hospital chains manage an additional 282 nonprofit hospitals with 35,000 beds.

The most striking for-profit hospital expansion has been the growth, largely by acquisition, of multihospital corporate chains. They operate about 11 percent of all U.S. community hospitals and 9 percent of the beds. One prediction plots their proportion at 20 percent by 1990, with revenues jumping from $13 billion in 1984 to $64 billion in 1990.

The four largest hospital chains, Hospital Corporation of America, Humana, American Medical International, and National Medical Enterprises, together owned 435 hospitals (including psychiatric and other special-purpose institutions), controlled more than half the for-profit beds, and had revenues of more than $10 billion in 1984. The Big Four chains also own and operate hospitals abroad in England, Switzerland, France, Spain, Saudi Arabia, and elsewhere.

For-profit chains tend to be diversified, particularly within the health industry. National Medical Enterprises owns 286 nursing homes and leases 21 more. It distributes hospital supplies, operates retail pharmacies, and sells building materials. American Medical International, concentrated in Texas and California, offers management and consulting services. Hospital Corporation of America owns 18 percent of Beverly Enterprises, the largest nursing-home chain, and in 1985 tried unsuccessfully to merge with American Hospital Supply Corporation, the nation's largest seller of medical supplies. Humana owns the largest chain of freestanding surgicenters that perform outpatient surgery, called Humana MedFirst. The Big Four are starting their own preferred provider organizations, which offer hospital care and an increasing range of outpatient services to large corporations at present charges. By the end of 1984, Humana had contracts with 200 companies covering 65,000 people.

For-profit hospitals seek the prestige and specialized services that come with facilities for medical research. Teaching and research centers also allow for-profit chains to provide all levels of care and to avoid sending patients outside their own systems for complex, expensive, and high-profit-margin procedures. In 1984 American Medical International bought St. Joseph Hospital in Omaha, a 539-bed Catholic teaching hospital of Creighton University, for $100 million. Hospital Corporation of America announced plans in 1984 to pay $265 million for the 760-bed Wesley Medical Center, a nonprofit research center in Wichita, Kansas. HCA also unsuccessfully attempted to buy a teaching hospital associated with Harvard University but backed off after faculty protests. Humana is leasing and managing the University of Louisville medical complex. Humana also hired Dr. William C. DeVries, guaranteed to underwrite 100 artificial heart operations at $250,000 each, and gained international attention with a series of implants.

With the decline in direct public spending for hospital construction and new equipment, for-profit chains have greater access to capital than most nonprofit hospitals. The for-profits can raise money through stock sales and a wide variety of debt instruments, including bank loans, Eurodollar financing, commercial paper, convertible debt, subordinated debentures, and industrial revenue bonds, as well as conventional mortgage financing. Hospital chains have been among the most highly leveraged industries in America, with debt constituting 60 to 85 percent of their capital structure.

Some evidence suggests that for-profit hospitals charge more than the nonprofits. The Congressional Office of Technology Assessment found that for-profit hospital chains generally increase the cost of care by providing more ancillary services and by higher markups on costs. A North Carolina Blue Cross/Blue Shield study found that "for-profit hospitals in the state generally charge significantly more than not-for-profit hospitals for the same operation." The higher charges were mainly for ancillary services: "pharmacy and medical/surgical supplies and to a lesser extent, operating room and anesthesia charges." The study concluded that charges in for-profit hospitals were 6 to 58 percent higher than in nonprofit hospitals of similar size. Three of four nonprofit hospitals sold to for-profit corporations raised their charges immediately after sale. One increased charges 113 percent in the first two years. During the same period, similar nonprofit hospitals increased their charges only a third as much. The American Federation of Hospitals, the for-profits' association, claims that the difference between costs and revenues is about the same for nonprofits and for-profits, just over 5 percent; but the return on equity for corporations such as Hospital Corporation of America has been two to three times as much.

There are also indications that for-profit hospitals, particularly chains, refuse to treat indigent and Medicaid patients. Mike Wallace, in a 1985 *60 Minutes* broadcast, exposed the billfold biopsies that for-profit hospitals like Dallas–Fort Worth Medical Center and Charter-Suburban perform in dumping patients without funds or insurance on Dallas's public hospital, Parkland. In this regard nonprofit chains appear to have a better, but hardly enviable, record. It is clear that, despite Medicare and Medicaid reimbursements, government-run public hospitals shoulder a disproportionate share of the burden of caring for patients without insurance or private funds. In 1983 the American Hospital Association reported that charity care and bad debts represented 11.5 percent of public hospitals' revenues, while accounting for only 4.2 percent of nonprofit hospitals' revenues and 3.1 percent of the revenues of for-profit hospitals. Charity care alone accounted for only one-tenth of 1 percent of for-profit hospital revenues, compared with 1.2 percent of nonprofit hospital revenues and 4.2 percent of public hospital revenues. The National Association of Public Hospitals calculates that public hospitals, with 20 percent of the beds, provide 43 percent of unpaid care; private nonprofit hospitals, with about 70 percent of the beds, provide just over 50 percent of unpaid care, and for-profits, with about 10 percent of the beds, provide less than 5 percent of the unpaid care.

The most troubling concerns stem from the danger that the profit motive—and the legal obligations to produce for stockholders—will undermine professional standards and reduce concern for social and individual problems. The debate over the role and regulation of for-profit hospitals is likely to intensify. They have been accused of limiting the number of uninsured and Medicaid patients they will take, reducing valuable but low-profit-margin services, maintaining unnecessarily high occupancy rates by assigning admitting percentages to doctors, and encouraging excessive use of ancillary services. Will profit-oriented hospitals seeking high occupancy rates pay too little attention to such unprofitable activities as health promotion, disease prevention, early detection, environmental and occupational safety? When big business comes to the bedside, what happens to the doctor-patient relationship?

Vertical mergers of hospitals with suppliers harbor the potential for serious conflicts of interest that could unnecessarily increase the risk and cost to the patient. As for-profit hospitals join hands with corporations who are inventing and selling expensive medical devices, can they keep the focus on both profit and patient at the same time? Should a corporation that owns hospitals, psychiatric units, HMOs, hospices, and/or home health care operations be allowed to own drug companies and medical equipment manufacturers? Or should such vertical integration be curtailed because of the conflicts it creates?

There is the deep concern that profit-making hospital and health care providers will keep their eyes fixed on profits—providing services that give the highest return, encouraging tests or services of high profit margin, directing patients to related suppliers, like pharmacies, eyeglass shops, or nursing homes, even if these are more expensive than other suppliers. Such attitudes are understandable in the operation of grocery or department stores. Are they acceptable in the health care arena? How do we get the substantial benefits of competition, efficiency, and variety from for-profit business activity and maintain the ethical standards appropriate for health care? Can we, as Michael Bromberg, executive director of the for-profit hospital association, argues, forge innovative contractual arrangements that will sustain high-quality care and medical research, and provide treatment of needy patients at for-profit hospitals? Or, as a team of researchers at Johns Hopkins University suggests, are the for-profit hospital corporations just interested in the prestige and high gross revenues of teaching facilities that improve a company's stock price and ability to attract capital?

As Dr. Arnold Relman, the editor of the *New England Journal of Medicine*, has put it, "Health care is not something you can sell and buy like a refrigerator or a pair of shoes. It's different. It's a social service." It has been relatively easy for the profiters to answer Relman and other critics in a fee-for-service, cost-based payment environment, where they have largely cashed in by creaming affluent sections of the nation and neighborhoods filled with well-insured private patients and Medicare beneficiaries. How the pressure for profits will coexist with humane and professional medicine is very much a question as for-profit hospital corporations face Medicare's diagnosis related groups, similar pressures from comparable private plans to reduce the cost of employee health care, and demands that they take on a fair share of indigent and Medicaid patients.

AFTER DIAGNOSIS RELATED GROUPS:
A REVOLUTION FOR HOSPITALS?

A central catalyst for change in the American hospital has been the payment system Medicare began introducing in October 1983. J. Alexander McMahon, head of the American Hospital Association, claims that "Medicare prospective pricing overshadows all other developments facing the hospital industry." Medicare accounts for almost 30 percent of hospital revenues. From the beginning, Medicare paid each hospital on the basis of its costs (with cost-plus factors in the case of for-profits). The maximum payments allowed were loosely related to average costs at similar hospitals. Thus, if similar hospitals were inefficient and expensive, the maximum went up. There was no reward for the efficient and no penalty for the profligate.

On October 1, 1983, under the gun from an uneasy Congress, Medicare adopted a prospective payment system for hospitals, to be phased in over three years. The system identifies 470 "diagnosis related groups" (DRGs) for different medical conditions, from heart attacks to broken bones. Medicare determines in advance what it will pay for each DRG. During the phase-in period, Medicare's payments are based on each hospital's own cost base for treatment and on regional and national costs. (When fully phased in, DRGs are expected to be based on a single national payment structure, reflecting urban-rural differences but not cost variations for individual hospitals.) The DRGs are designed to cover most major variations in need for care, based on the diagnoses, surgical procedures, sex and age of the patient at admission, and complications, if any. For instance, there are four separate DRGs for an appendectomy, taking into account whether the patient is more than sixty-nine years old and whether complications exist.

See what this does to the hospitals' economic incentives. DRGs pay a certain amount for each Medicare patient admitted with a particular diagnosis, no matter how long the stay or how many services rendered. If a hospital spends more on a Medicare patient than the DRG rate, it loses money. However, if it spends less than the DRG rate, it makes money. Thus the hospital's incentives are reversed. No longer does Medicare pay more for more services or pick up the bill on a cost or cost-plus basis.

To discourage hospitals from inappropriately admitting patients or providing too little care, Congress told Medicare to establish peer review organizations (PROs) across the country, composed of doctors, other providers, and consumers. By the end of 1984, virtually all of the fifty-four areas so designated had PRO contracts with Medicare. The PROs' responsibilities are to ensure that there is no skimping on care and to eliminate unnecessary admissions and hospital days. These organizations have the power to prevent admissions under Medicare for elective surgery and to block payments for unnecessary services. They have committed themselves to lower Medicare expenditures by reducing unnecessary admissions and hospital services.

Wisconsin's PRO (WIPRO), for example, has set objectives that would provide a net savings to the government (after paying WIPRO) of $14 million over two years and cut Medicare's Wisconsin expenditures by 1 percent. The Columbia, South Carolina, PRO plans to reduce Medicare admissions by 50 percent, largely by encouraging outpatient care. The Indiana Medical Review Organization in Terre Haute expects to reduce inappropriate admissions by 3,100 in just twelve DRGs. The Empire State Medical, Scientific, and Educational Foundation PRO in Lake Success, New York, found that less than half of the 24,560 colonoscopies performed in 1982 helped physicians make a diagnosis. In the first months of its review process, the New York PRO disallowed 14 percent of the Medicare payments to New York City hospitals because of inappropriate admissions and excessive lengths of stay.

These PROs may prove critical to effective operation of the DRG system. Some physicians, like Dr. John Wennberg of Dartmouth and Dr. Philip Caper of Harvard, have warned that the DRG pressures for prompt release of hospital patients could encourage doctors and hospitals to increase the number of hospital admissions in order to keep beds filled. Some increases could be accomplished within accepted medical standards because of the enormous variations in medical practice.

The danger of prematurely releasing a patient is also present in a system that pays the same amount whether hospitalization lasts two or ten days. Investigations in 1985 by the General Accounting Office, the Department of Health and Human Services, and the Senate Special Committee on Aging suggest that some Medicare patients are being discharged too soon, or erroneously told to leave because their benefits are exhausted. These patients end up in what Senator John Heinz of Pennsylvania calls a "no-care" zone, where nursing homes reject them because the homes are full or the patients are too sick. PROs must pursue cases of inadequate care as aggressively as they attack cases of excessive care.

No regulatory system is immune from manipulation, and the DRG system does provide a temptation to maximize payment. A hospital can interpret complications so as to assign patients to the highest-paying DRGs. This was a problem early on in New Jersey, which first adopted a DRG system in 1980.

In developing the DRG rates for medical complications, Medicare had anticipated some "DRG creep," i.e., that more high-cost cases would be reported than in the past, because of better hospital record-keeping and manipulation of the system. However, the first nine months of the program saw hospitals reporting high-cost cases far exceeding Medicare's generous predictions. To compensate for unwarranted DRG creep, Medicare proposed to reduce the value of the complication weights by 2.4 percent in setting fiscal 1985 schedules.

The hospital industry objected, claiming that the big DRG creep simply reflected the fact that they were treating sicker patients. It flexed its political muscle with Congress and the White House. To put heat on Medicare, the Senate Finance Subcommittee on Health held a hastily scheduled special hearing just three months before the 1984 elections. The White House put the arm on the Department of Health and Human Services. On August 29, 1984, two months before the election, Medicare backed down and reduced the weights by less than half its original proposal. The adjustment in the hospital's favor cost taxpayers at least $350 million in fiscal 1985. The Congress also bowed to hospital pressures to boost DRG rates above Medicare's proposal in 1985—despite record-breaking hospital profits in 1984 and early 1985 and revelations by the Department of Health and Human Services that hospital profits on Medicare patients hit $5 billion in 1984, a 14 percent margin, three times the average profit on all patients in the early 1980s.

Despite these political hassles, the DRG system is off to a good start in reducing costs. For the 5,405 hospitals operating under DRGs in 1984, the average length of stay for Medicare patients dropped from 9.5 to 7.4 days. Nationally, average length of stay for all patients sixty-five and over has dropped from 9.7 to 8.9 days. In 1984 admissions of patients over sixty-four were down 2.9 percent from a year earlier. As a result, Medicare hospital expenditures were $2.2 billion below budget projections.

Keeping people out of the hospital not only saves money, it saves lives. In 1983, an estimated 1.9 million hospital patients acquired new diseases while in the hospital and 96,000 died from causes related to these new diseases. In 1984, when there were 1.5 million fewer hospital admissions, an estimated 75,000 fewer patients got sick in the hospital and 3,700 fewer died.

The ripple effects of DRGs, an aroused business community, and states fighting their own cost-control battles combined to further change the environment for hospitals. Reductions in lengths of stay and 1 million fewer admissions for the under-sixty-five population, along with the DRG payment system, reduced 1984 hospital bed occupancy rates to 5.6 percent below those of the previous year. Many hospitals were less than 60 percent occupied. Employment in community hospitals, which had increased steadily for twenty years, declined in 1984, and some hospitals for the first time in memory laid off employees and imposed pay cuts.

After ten years of annual profit increases of 20 percent among the for-profit hospitals, the largest chain, Hospital Corporation of America, announced that its 1985 fourth-quarter profits would be flat, and that 1986 profits would not exceed 1985's. Stunned by 49 percent occupancy rates, HCA cut its hospital acquisition budget in half and announced a strategy of buying health insurance companies. American Medical International revealed that its 1985 fourth-quarter (ending September 30) net income had dropped 38 percent, as actions by business and government slashed occupancy rates.

Blue Cross/Blue Shield, the nation's largest health insurer, offered the federal government and 1.5 million of its employees a $754 million refund of health insurance premiums for 1984. This was made possible by an unprecedented 22 percent decline between 1983 and 1984 in the total number of days policyholders spent in the hospital.

To make up for lost business in admissions and lengths of stay, hospitals are aggressively soliciting doctors to get more patients. In California, Hollywood Community Hospital, part of a for-profit chain, has offered to share its DRG payments with doctors when their patients' bills are more than 75 percent reimbursed by Medicare. (The AMA has condemned such payments as kickbacks.) For-profit hospital companies are going directly to corporations, offering special discounts and preferred provider arrangements, including outpatient care and administration of claims. Hospitals are adding services such as urgent care centers, alcohol treatment programs, ambulatory care, nursing homes, rehabilitation centers, primary care centers, birthing centers, wellness centers, occupational health programs, sports medicine clinics, and sleeping and eating disorder programs. By one estimate, in 1990 hospitals will collect more than $5 billion annually for services such as these.

Hospitals are also diversifying. By 1984, 25 percent were providing home health care and another 35 percent planned to get into that business. To the extent that this far less costly care replaces expensive days in the hospital, total health costs will be reduced.

Hospitals have gone to Madison Avenue to help them develop new markets. In 1983 health care professionals, led by hospitals, spent $41 million on television spots, up more than eleven times from 1977's $3.7 million. In 1985, hospitals employed two thousand marketing executives, compared with six in 1978. Illinois Masonic Medical Center in Chicago advertised 25 percent reductions in rates for semiprivate rooms; Greater Southeast Community Hospital in Washington, D.C., ran radio ads, complete with a catchy musical jingle, hawking reduced rates for "comfortable homelike rooms" and "overnight guest" privileges. Hospitals now advertise rebates to patients who have to wait more than a few minutes in an emergency room, or those whose floor nurses do not answer a call within one or two minutes.

Methodist Medical Center in Illinois provides valet parking. Southwood Community Hospital in Norfolk, Massachusetts, saturated its community with direct mail brochures that enclosed coupons for a free medical encyclopedia for those who patronized the hospital's walk-in clinic. St. Joseph's Hospital in Flint, Michigan, lured patients with a widely advertised "Special Delivery" package: for the expectant mother, a twenty-four-hour hospital stay with follow-up visits for only $799—less than a third of the regular delivery cost of up to $3,000. Deliveries rose from 1,200 to 1,650 in the first year.

It's too soon to tell whether the softening of the hospital business is a pause to catch breath in the twenty-year marathon of escalating costs, or whether a new era of efficiency is at hand. The slower increase in hospital costs largely reflects reduced utilization. Even with the overall lessening of inflationary pressures in the economy, in 1984 the price of hospital services rose at twice the rate of the consumer price index and in some states, like Michigan, continued to rise at a double-digit pace. And despite fewer admissions and shorter lengths of stay, hospitals overall recorded greater profits (surpluses) in 1984 than ever before, and 1985 first-quarter profits were up 22 percent, heralding another record-breaking year.

Hospitals responded temporarily to the threat of cost containment in 1978 and 1979, when, as Secretary of HEW, I tried to get legislation through Congress to limit the rate of increase in hospital charges; when the bill failed, the high increases in rates resumed. Hospitals have also demonstrated repeatedly that they know how to pull the political strings to make the Medicare system work for them. Their original reluctant embrace of Medicare became a torrid affair as the hospital lobby tailored the system to their interests.

Will DRGs suffer the same fate? It's too soon to tell, but the limits of government regulation over an industry with the money and power of hospitals and doctors are clear.

The test for us—as employers, employees, insurers, and most of all, citizens, consumers, and patients—is to give hospitals the right mix of rewards and penalties to motivate them to care about cost as well as service. Whether we're smart enough and tough enough to do that may well determine whether there is a first-class health care system for our children.

Chapter 7

THE PROFITABLE
ACOLYTES

The hard core of the health industry—the doctors, dentists, allied health professionals, and hospitals—has spawned an array of profitable acolytes. There are insurance companies to plot the odds, handle the paperwork, and pay the bills; pharmaceutical companies to invent, patent, and market drugs; equipment manufacturers to make prostheses, artificial hearts, and machines that help diagnose disease; biotechnology companies that may revolutionize medical care with the fruits of recombinant DNA (deoxyribonucleic acid) research.

By and large, these acolytes have made money. They have benefited enormously from the fee-for-service and cost-based third-party reimbursement systems that characterized health care payments until 1984. But this could change. They are no longer settled as comfortably leeward of the winds of competition as they were in the 1970s and early 1980s.

THE HEALTH INSURERS

The commercial insurance companies and the Blues are the money changers, particularly in the temples of hospital care. While no one is about to drive them out, they are under increasing pressure to represent the interests of the patients they insure rather than the suppliers whose bills they collect. For the first time in their history, the health insurers and the Blues are being pressed hard to respond to the big customers who pay their bills—the large corporate employers. It's none too soon.

The largest commercial health insurer, Prudential, with assets of more than $80 billion in 1984, took in almost $3 billion in health insurance premiums that year. Aetna Life Insurance Company, Travelers Insurance Company, and Connecticut General Life Insurance Company each got more than $2 billion in health insurance premiums. Mutual of Omaha Insurance Company received more than $1.6 billion.

While the largest twenty commercial insurers do 50 percent of the business and tend to set the pace, more than 1,000 commercial companies sell health insurance. Most of the big commercial health insurers cut their teeth in the life and property insurance business. But insuring health is a more dicey business than insuring life. Benefit payments are volatile, influenced by rising medical costs, inflation rates, hospital utilization, changes in the population insured, enrollments, and the services covered. In periods of unexpectedly high inflation, medical costs can be substantially higher than estimates used to calculate premiums. As unemployment rises, workers facing layoffs take advantage of benefits they fear they'll lose if they are laid off. To protect themselves and ensure profits, insurers rarely set premiums beyond one year. In 1984 commercial insurers collected $43.6 billion in premiums and paid only $33.3 billion in claims, 76 cents per premium dollar. The amount of claims paid for each premium dollar has been dropping steadily since 1981.

As health care has become a large part of the cost of doing business, insurance has changed. Most large corporations have created some kind of self-funded health plan for their employees, in which the "premiums" remain with the company and the company pays the bills; a health insurer processes the claims and does the paperwork, in what have become known as "administrative service only" plans. Often, the corporation will also buy insurance against large, unpredictable claims that its reserves might not be able to handle. These kinds of plans constituted some 30 percent of group coverage in 1984, up sixfold from 1975.

In addition to commercial insurers, there are 88 Blue Cross and Blue Shield plans: Blue Cross for hospital expenses and Blue Shield for physicians' and surgeons' fees. These plans, frequently operated jointly, are organized in each state and in some metropolitan areas. The plans belong to a national association, which provides research, statistical, actuarial, marketing, and lobbying services, and helps coordinate health care coverage for some large national employers. The Blues have been organized on a nonprofit basis, but in 1985 Congress began a move to lift their tax-exempt status.

In 1984 the Blues as a group registered a surplus in their underwriting operations, receiving $39.9 billion in premiums and paying out about $35.7 billion in claims. After expenses, they had a net gain of nearly $1 billion from subscriptions plus another $1 billion from investment and other income, which produced more than $2 billion in additional reserves in 1984 to carry over to 1985 as a cushion against increased charges.

Together, the commercial insurers, the Blues, and the self-insured corporations provide widely varying kinds of insurance coverage to about 175 million Americans. Many people are covered by more than one policy, and many are covered for only part of a year. Virtually all have some sort of hospitalization coverage, including about 50 million through HMOs, fraternal and community organizations, cooperatives, and plans administered directly by employers or labor unions. The total number of people with hospital and surgical coverage has grown steadily but slowly since 1977 at 1.5 to 2 percent per year, with a slight dip in 1981 as unemployment rates rose. But the Blues' share of the market has been steadily declining. Since 1950 the Blues coverage of individuals with hospitalization insurance has slipped from 50 to just over 40 percent.

As with so much of the health care industry, the health insurance business is in turmoil. There has been competition among insurers for some time, but insurers are now vying with hospital chains and clinics, HMOs, and preferred providers that offer services (including claims administration) directly to big corporations, and with former big customers that self-insure. Of special significance, over the long haul, is the changing relationship between insurers and government and corporate purchasers of insurance and administrative services, who are insisting that the insurance industry act as their agents.

Until the 1980s, the Blues and the commercial insurers—despite their occasional protestations and marketing rhetoric—acted as though their bread was buttered by health care suppliers, notably the doctors and hospitals, paying them whatever they charged. Indeed, the congressional decision in 1965 to allow hospitals to select the intermediaries (health insurance companies) who would process their Medicare claims gave a legislative nod to the cozy relationship between insurers and doctors and hospitals.

Two incidents during my tenure as Secretary of HEW point up the problem in this arrangement. In 1977 I was appalled to discover the extent to which the commercial insurers and Blues, who were supposed to be protecting the public interest in administering Medicare (and to some extent Medicaid), were hired guns for hospitals and doctors. I moved on two fronts: to seek competitive bids from companies who wanted to make money administering Medicare claims and to end the suppliers' control over the Blues.

To solicit competitive bids, I invoked the Secretary's authority to conduct demonstrations in search of more efficient ways to operate. The results were amazing: bidders offered to process Medicare claims in the future at a charge per claim less than half of what HEW was paying to insurance companies and Blues selected by hospitals. Moreover, the bidders indicated far more willingness to help HEW police the hospitals, doctors, and pharmacists.

What did the Blues do? They sued—unsuccessfully—to enjoin me from awarding these bids or going out on any others. (They did prevail, however, in blocking my efforts to have the law amended to permit competitive bidding as a routine matter.)

This reaction of the Blues heightened my concern that their boards were so dominated by providers, mainly doctors and hospital administrators, that they were unable to represent the interests of the consumer, government or private. This was particularly true of Blue Shield: twenty of the thirty-two plans administering Medicare claims for physician payments had boards with 50 percent or more provider membership. I announced my intention to develop a regulation that would require the boards of Blue Cross and Blue Shield to have a majority of members who were not providers of health care. Even though the national Blue Cross Association had already begun requiring majority public membership on boards of its member plans, you would have thought I was trying to give a parched boy a glass of old-fashioned castor oil and vinegar to quench his thirst. The Blues declared war on the regulation, took their case to their friends on Capitol Hill, and prevented the issuance of a final order for the duration of my time in office. Although no regulation was ever issued, by 1982 the Blues had voluntarily, if reluctantly, adopted policies requiring nonprovider majorities on their boards.

These battles helped break up the intimate relationship between the commercial insurers and Blues and the doctors and hospitals. The metamorphosis of the insurers into energetic advocates of those who pay the bills is likely to be achieved in the private sector, motivated particularly by big business. In 1984 more and more corporations insisted that their insurer—commercial or Blues, whether acting as the insurer or just administering a self-insured plan—represent their interests. The big companies are demanding that their group insurers review health care utilization patterns, monitor physicians and hospitals, and discipline those providers who exceed standards established for reasonable testing, drug prescriptions, admissions, or lengths of stay. If the commercial insurers and the Blues want to keep their corporate business, they're beginning to realize, they must respond to those who pay their bills. Indeed, the perception of the Blues as agents of doctors and hospitals has been responsible in good measure for the decline in their market share.

There is real evidence of change. Seventy-five percent of the large commercial insurers in 1984 reimbursed patients for second opinions for nonemergency surgery, compared with just 14 percent a decade earlier. In 1982, Blue Cross greatly expanded a modest cost-control program begun in the late 1970s, issuing guidelines to stop unnecessary respiratory treatment in hospitals. Respiratory therapies are among the fastest-growing hospital procedures. They have been administered to 25 percent of all hospital patients at an annual cost of $4 billion. One procedure—intermittent positive-pressure breathing (IPPB), a mechanical process to expand the lung—costs $1 billion each year. Blue Cross announced its plans not to pay for such therapy, often routinely given as part of the preoperative hospital testing, unless warranted by special circumstances, such as a known pulmonary problem or a history of smoking.

Another example is the push to limit the use of ultrasound machines, which project sound waves at a patient and create a television picture based on the echoes. Ultrasound is a valuable tool when used properly—for example, when a delivery is expected to pose problems—and unnecessarily expensive when used indiscriminately—for example, in all pregnancies. In 1984, Blue Cross/Blue Shield and several commercial insurers stopped reimbursing doctors and patients for use of ultrasound devices in routine pregnancies.

The Blues and most commercial insurers (and some private employers) now insist that many tests be run before the patient is admitted to the hospital. Plans with such preadmission testing have reported savings ranging from $400,000 to $1.7 million in a single year. Blue Cross and Blue Shield of Iowa estimate that their program saves 1,900 inpatient days annually; it helped them to reduce premiums in 1984. Insurance companies participating in the federal government's health program reduced premiums for 1986 by 6 percent because claims fell as much as 20 percent in the first nine months of 1985, the first drop in the program's twenty-five years.

THE DRUG INDUSTRY

Perhaps the most profitable acolytes are the pharmaceutical companies. These companies make a major contribution to good health and cost containment. Polio vaccination saves $90 for each $1 spent and has almost eliminated our most feared childhood disease, reducing it to seven new cases in 1984. Mumps and measles vaccination saves $14 for each $1 spent.

The industry is well paid for its work. In 1984 Americans spent $26 billion directly for drugs and medical sundries. We spent almost 60 percent of these dollars on prescriptions, 30 percent for over-the-counter preparations like Tylenol and cough syrup, and just over 10 percent for sundries, like Band-Aids, iodine, petroleum jelly, thermometers, and arch supports. If we add the cost of drugs dispensed by hospitals, nursing homes, physicians, and dentists, the total rises to about $38 billion, just about 1 percent of the gross national product, well over $150 for each man, woman, and child.

In 1984, Americans took 77 billion prescription pills and other drugs, making us the most drug-happy population in the world. Each year, Americans consume about 5 billion tranquilizers and sedatives. Each day, millions of Americans take a tranquilizer, like Librium or Valium. Each night millions take a pill to sleep.

As drugs are increasingly used to treat chronic diseases or their symptoms, or to prevent cardiovascular diseases, the numbers can only go up. By 1984, 60 percent of prescriptions were for chronic therapy.

Cardiovascular drugs accounted for some 13 percent of the total number of prescriptions in 1984, and with a new generation of drugs to treat angina and hypertension—calcium and beta blockers—their share is likely to grow. In the first year following its introduction in 1982, doctors wrote more than 4 million prescriptions for Pfizer's calcium blocker, Procardia. In 1983 Inderal, American Home Products' beta blocker, was the most prescribed drug in America, and Dyazide, a diuretic for hypertension made by SmithKline Beckman, was second.

Antibiotics and psychotropics each account for about 8 percent of prescription drugs sold; tranquilizers and painkillers like Valium, 7 percent; cold and cough prescriptions, about 6 percent; and antiarthritics, about 4 percent. Because virtually all antiarthritics are still on exclusive patent, this 4 percent of prescriptions represents 8 percent of the dollar value of pharmaceuticals sold.

Generic drugs, the therapeutic chemical equivalents of products on which the patents have expired, are an increasing proportion of prescription drugs manufactured by the big companies. In 1975 they represented 9.5 percent of the value of drugs sold; in 1983 they accounted for 20 percent. Generics are predicted to jump to more than 30 percent of prescription sales by 1990. They sell for 20 to 90 percent less than the brand name originals, and force reductions in the price of those originals. In 1984 Upjohn Company slashed 35 percent off the price of Motrin, an anti-inflammatory drug used to treat arthritis, in the face of competition from a generic equivalent.

In addition to buying prescription drugs, in 1984 Americans spent an estimated $8.4 billion on some 60,000 over-the-counter products. Painkillers account for about 29 percent of these sales; cough and cold items, 23 percent; digestive aids and antacids, 21 percent, and vitamins, 18 percent. An ongoing Food and Drug Administration review of over-the-counter products—which by 1984 had amassed 1,400 volumes of data—has found that some 250 were unsafe or ineffective and another 240 were of questionable value.

The profits of the drug companies are the envy of other industries. America's pharmaceutical corporations account for about one-quarter of the world's prescription and over-the-counter drugs. Although some 750 firms produce and sell drugs, 16 command two-thirds of the market. These are firms like American Home Products, with 1984 sales of $4.8 billion; Pfizer and Bristol-Myers, each with 1984 sales of $4 billion; Warner-Lambert, Merck & Company, SmithKline Beckman, and Eli Lilly, each with 1984 sales of $3 billion or more. G. D. Searle, Squibb, Sterling Drug, Upjohn, Schering-Plough, and Richardson-Vicks had 1984 sales in excess of $1 billion. *Fortune* magazine listed American Home Products, SmithKline Beckman, and Merck among the 13 most profitable companies during the decade 1974–1983.

Forbes magazine's 1984 "Annual Report of American Industry" showed the drug industry's median net profit margin as 10.6 percent, more than three times the median net profit for all U.S. industries. Only the electric utility industry enjoys a better median net profit. But *Forbes'* estimate may be low. *Value Line*, an investment analysis service, reported 1984 net profits industry-wide at 11.7 percent. A U.S. House of Representatives subcommittee on health reported in 1985 that after-tax profits of pharmaceutical companies averaged 12.7 percent from 1981 to 1984. Some firms have net profit projections substantially higher, such as Merck at 13.8 percent, American Home Products at 14.6 percent, Lilly at 15.5 percent, and SmithKline Beckman at 17 percent.

Drug companies argue that high profits are necessary because of the expense of developing a new drug (which can be as much as $50 million to $100 million) and to make up for losses on non-starters. Drug companies point out that 10 to 12 percent of their sales price is devoted to research and development. They spend nearly twice as much on advertising. The big advertising and promotion bucks are targeted at doctors—and with good effect for the drug companies. Two-thirds of all visits to doctors end with the patient walking out with a prescription. Thirty percent of those visits end with four or more prescriptions. Women get the lion's share of prescriptions: 60 percent. Senior citizens average eleven prescriptions a year. The drug companies have also expanded their advertising efforts beyond the doctors. Pfizer, for instance, has run a television ad encouraging overweight people over forty to get checked for diabetes. Concurrently, sales of Pfizer's Diabinese, a diabetic drug, jumped 15.4 percent. Other subjects of ad campaigns include hypertension drugs. Before the FDA imposed a moratorium in 1983 on advertising of specific prescription drugs directly to the public, one company was offering $1.50 coupons in bottles of its antiarthritic drug and another was pushing its pneumonia vaccine in magazine advertisements.

Advertising can sell ineffective drugs as well as effective ones. A twenty-two-year FDA study finished in 1984 found that of 3,443 prescription drugs examined, almost one-third—some 1,100—were not proved to be effective. As a result, the drugs have been removed from the market. Another 7,000 similar drugs were modified or prohibited from sale. But not before billions of pills were sold for billions of dollars to millions of Americans, unnecessarily increasing our health costs and risks.

Drug prices reflect their status in the third-party health care reimbursement system. Unlike virtually all hospital and most doctor bills, bills for drugs are ordinarily paid directly by the consumer. Individuals pay some 79 percent of drug bills, with private health insurance paying only 12 percent and government programs only 9 percent. So drug pricing tends to be more reflective of the general marketplace, particularly when patents have expired.

Although drug prices have gone up threefold since 1972, for most of that period increases averaged about 9 percent a year, less than the increase in the overall consumer price index and far less than the rises in hospital charges. From 1981 to mid-1985, however, pharmaceutical prices shot up at more than twice the rate of increase in the CPI. Prescription drug prices climbed at 56 percent versus 23 percent for the CPI, as newly patented drugs became a physician-preferred treatment for chronic heart disease and arthritis.

Patented drugs command high prices, especially when only one patented drug will work on a particular disease. The antiulcer drug Tagamet, with 1982 sales at nearly $1 billion worldwide, is reported to produce one-half of SmithKline Beckman's profits. At the peak of its exclusive patent, Motrin, an antiarthritic drug, is said to have provided about one-third of Upjohn's earnings. The tranquilizers Librium and Valium kept the profit coffers overflowing at Hoffmann–La Roche, and antibiotics delivered handsome profits to a number of drug companies for many years.

But once the cocoon of the patent is peeled off, drug prices reflect the marketplace—not the health care marketplace. That's why the pharmaceutical giants fought so hard for legislation to extend the seventeen-year patent period to take account of Food and Drug Administration delays in clearing drugs for use. Passed in 1984, this legislation permits drug makers to extend the patent life of products up to five years, to compensate for the time elapsed between the date of the original patent and completion of Food and Drug Administration review and approval, a lapse that manufacturers claimed had cut the useful patent life of drug products from seventeen years to an average of seven years.

The profit potential of an extra five years of patent protection is so great that the drug companies were willing to relax their opposition to speeding up the availability of generic drugs after patent expiration. The same bill that increased patent protection authorized a stepped-up procedure to approve generic copies of drugs. As a result, generics will be far more quickly available to the public after the original patents expire. By late 1985, just ten months after the legislation became effective, the FDA had received 650 applications for approval of generic drugs and had approved generic substitutes for nine of the ten top-selling prescription drugs, including Valium. Production of at least 200 generic substitutes is expected to be stimulated by 1987, saving consumers and government purchasers millions of dollars.

American businesses, especially the big corporate purchasers of health insurance, are likely to become the most aggressive promoters of generic drugs, providing economic incentives for their employees to insist upon the less expensive generic equivalents of brand name drugs, as a part of their cost-control strategies. Not surprisingly, the major pharmaceutical companies are increasingly manufacturing these generic substitutes.

Drugs such as calcium and beta blockers, which should reduce demand for bypass surgery, can be quite cost-effective. But drugs can also stoke the high-tech fires of supersurgery. Since the early 1980s, cyclosporin has greatly increased the ability of patients to accept vital-organ transplants. A year's supply of this drug, which transplant patients take for the rest of their lives, can cost as much as $18,000.

Drug companies need help to continue to produce vaccines against childhood diseases (and possibly flu vaccines for people over sixty-five and high-risk individuals of all ages). The childhood vaccination program is perhaps the most cost-effective medical enterprise in America, to say nothing of the pain, suffering, life-long disability, and human anguish it averts. Yet some vaccines, particularly DPT—diphtheria, pertussis (whooping cough), tetanus—carry a risk of severe reaction. For DPT and other childhood vaccines, the risk is statistically tiny, but the potential liability (particularly for pain and emotional distress) is such that it hikes the price enormously—DPT vaccine cost twenty times as much in 1984 as it did in 1982—and threatens pharmaceutical company balance sheets. As a result, companies are reluctant to manufacture the vaccines. By the beginning of 1985, we had only two manufacturers of DPT vaccine, and only one producer each of other vaccines, such as those for measles and polio. As Secretary of HEW, I warned of this problem, and by 1984 the Department of Health and Human Services had begun stockpiling vaccines for fear that the manufacturers might stop producing them. We need a permanent solution, one that sufficiently eases the liability of the drug companies in return for their agreement to manufacture these childhood vaccines; that maintains high standards of care in production and distribution; and that encourages drug companies to search for even safer vaccines. Any number of alternatives are available; the government should adopt one promptly.

There is precedent for assisting the drug industry in the federal government's assumption of liability for certain adverse reactions to swine flu vaccine in the 1970s, in California's immunization reaction program, and in legislation Congress passed on orphan drugs. These drugs hold the potential to cure diseases that afflict relatively small numbers of people, such as Huntington's disease and myoclonus. Congress defined an orphan drug as one useful in treating a disease affecting fewer than 200,000 persons in the United States, or one whose manufacturer has no expectation of recovering the costs of development and distribution. The act authorized seven years of exclusive marketing rights for orphan drugs that are not patentable, and streamlined the approval process by requiring the FDA to tell a manufacturer in advance exactly what tests would be necessary to get its okay to sell the drug. The bill authorized grants to manufacturers and others for clinical trials of designated drugs, and tax credits worth $15 million per year.

HIGHTECHNOPHILIA:
MEDICAL EQUIPMENT AND SUPPLIES

The value of medical and dental instruments and supplies manufactured in this country hit $20 billion in 1984. The medical equipment and supply industry produces some 130,000 products, from multimillion-dollar nuclear scanners and medical lasers to one-cent cotton swabs and tongue depressors. Of the hundreds of firms in each of the four major categories—X-ray and electromedical equipment, surgical instruments, surgical appliances, and dental equipment—four companies account for more than 30 percent of sales.

Within this industry, the most spectacular high-growth area has been in sophisticated diagnostic equipment, CAT, MR, and PET scanners and ultrasonic devices. General Electric, Johnson and

Johnson, Diasonics, Phillips, Seimens A.G., GEC/Picker, Intermagnetics General, and Fonar Corporation are among the big players in these markets. General Electric estimates that the domestic market for MRs alone will reach $630 million in 1987. Medicare's decision in 1985 to cover MR scans—which officials said was pressed more by lawyers and investment bankers than by doctors and patients—is central to GE's sales projections.

Although analysts of the medical equipment and supply industry are bullish on specific technologies, cost-consciousness is clouding the industry's profit outlook. As admissions and lengths of stay have decreased, hospitals are cautious about making large purchases and are far more price-conscious about the supplies and equipment they do buy. The signals are there, particularly in pressures on hospitals to use expensive technology sparingly. The increased vigilance of health insurers and large purchasers of care is tightening reimbursement for use of expensive diagnostic tools, limiting payment to need-to-use situations, with health insurers no longer hesitant about second-guessing doctors and hospitals. This tightfisted approach has had its effect on the medical supply companies: instead of its annual double-digit rate of increase for ten years, Baxter-Travenol revenues were down 2.3 percent in 1984; at American Hospital Supply, revenues increased only 4.2 percent compared with 11.6 percent in 1983; other medical supply manufacturers, like Johnson and Johnson and Becton Dickinson, showed only slight revenue gains in 1984.

A measure of the pressure from American business to rein in medical technology can be gleaned from its criticism of the Medicare DRG system. The reimbursement system includes in each DRG payment an automatic percentage to cover the cost of new equipment. The Washington Business Group on Health considers this a loophole and opposes any such percentage increase in DRG rates for new technology: "Advances must be economically efficient over their life cycle. No other industry receives a future price increase guarantee for technology, and medicine should not be an exception."

Properly used, expensive technology can save money as well as improve health. In late 1984 the Food and Drug Administration approved a new device, the $1.7 million lithotripter, which uses shock waves to pulverize kidney stones, eliminating the need for painful operations. This device could save money by rendering most operations to remove kidney stones unnecessary—if purchasers of health care insist on its efficient use, and Medicare's DRG system and corporate insurers give hospitals the will to resist the temptation to acquire such a machine simply to keep up with the neighbors. The cost-containment omens are not good. The maximum estimated need for the entire country is 100 lithotripters. By mid-1985, hospitals had installed 14 and ordered another 150.

Proper use—particularly avoiding unnecessary use—is essential to getting medical technology to work efficiently for better health. More than 500,000 pacemakers have been installed in Americans, and 130,000 are expected to be installed each year, at $4,000 apiece. These devices offer the patient years of productive life when properly used. But the Health Research Group investigated more than 2,000 pacemaker implants in Maryland and found at least 500 unnecessary and more than 280 questionable, at a cost of $3.5 million and risk for hundreds of human beings.

Medical equipment inventors and manufacturers face increased surveillance by the FDA. Like new drugs, new equipment technologies sometimes have bugs—fatal bugs. For instance, a 1984 FDA memorandum estimated that a mechanical heart valve implanted in thousands of people since 1979 may have resulted in as many as 320 deaths owing to a faulty weld. The Food and Drug Administration, after delaying action on a proposal started through the bureaucratic process in the late 1970s, issued a rule in September 1984 requiring manufacturers and importers of some 11,000 medical devices to report deaths and serious injuries resulting from their use. The FDA acknowledged that this rule would have given the early warning necessary to deal with problems in a new anesthesia machine that resulted in four deaths. Like all innovative medical procedures, use of new devices carries some risk.

BIOTECHNOLOGY:
HOW EXPENSIVE A BRAVE NEW WORLD?

Biotechnology, bioengineering, recombinant DNA research, cloning, gene-splicing—the exotica of medical technology—all make

Huxley's Brave New World a lot more real than anyone in the early 1930s imagined it could become. And they make it a lot harder to distinguish between Madame Curie and Dr. Frankenstein. Standard and Poor's estimates that some 10,000 laboratories in universities, government agencies, and private and public organizations around the world are involved in genetic engineering research. More than 200 companies market biotechnological products. With only a handful of commercial successes, the biotechnology industry raised more than $2.5 billion in capital in its first decade.

It's an exciting world, with unlimited potential. Recombinant DNA technology, central to many new products, involves removing genes from the DNA of one organism and inserting them in the DNA of another. The new genetic structure can then reproduce itself, exhibiting the hereditary qualities of the donor gene.

One of the first commercially viable products from genetic technology was a human insulin developed by Genentech. Introduced in 1982, it can be used by people allergic to animal insulin and it is easier to produce. Eli Lilly, which manufactures and markets the product as Humulin, saw sales climb from $10 million in 1983 to an estimated $25 million in 1984.

The first human vaccine created through recombinant DNA technology is expected to be on the market by 1987. Developed by Merck & Company, the vaccine created hepatitis B antibodies without harmful side effects in tests on Merck volunteers.

Monoclonal antibodies are used increasingly to detect pregnancy, particular cancers, and viruses, and may even be used in cancer treatment to carry anticancer radiation to tumor sites in the body. Other new diagnostic techniques, known as DNA probes, are under development.

The potential cost-effectiveness of these discoveries (not to mention ethical and safety issues in creating new forms of life) is likely to be scrutinized in a way that medical devices never were in the early years. Dr. Arnold Relman, editor of the *New England Journal of Medicine*, has charged that $5 billion to $10 billion a year is wasted on useless or dangerous medical technologies that, once put in hospitals or doctors' offices, must be used to pay their costs. The hardheadedness of big insurers, prodded by corporate purchasers of health care and the government's concern with cost containment, may make biotechnology the first health technology market that has to meet tests of cost-effectiveness and answer Harvard president Bok's question about the value of a human life.

Chapter 8

THE GOVERNMENT MONEY TREES

Medicare and Medicaid are the biggest money trees in the health care forest. Billions of dollars also sprout from the Defense Department, Veterans Administration, and National Institutes of Health, as well as from states and cities—but Medicare and Medicaid are the megahealth programs of government, providing the most dollars for America's health industry.

MEDICARE

In its first full year, 1967, Medicare cost $4.7 billion, less than 3 percent of the federal budget, to cover 19 million people. Since then, costs have jumped an average of 17 percent a year, even more sharply than the average yearly rise in total national health costs. In 1984 Medicare spent some $65 billion, picking up more than half of the federal government's $112 billion in health bills, gobbling up more than 7 percent of the entire federal budget to cover more than 30 million people (27 million senior citizens and 3 million disabled people).

By 1984 Medicare had become a bonanza for hospitals and medical equipment manufacturers, as 10 percent of its dollars paid for expensive, frequently high-tech care for beneficiaries with less than a month to live, and more than 30 percent paid for such care for those with less than a year. Medicare covers about 74 percent of its beneficiaries' hospital bills, and about 55 percent of their

doctors' bills. It is the second-largest domestic program, after Social Security. By 1990 Medicare costs will nudge $150 billion.

Medicare's role as pacesetter is not surprising since it is the largest single source of income for many health care providers. In 1984
Medicare provided hospitals almost 30 percent of their revenues
and doctors 21 percent of theirs. Some specialists get an even
higher share of their income from Medicare: thoracic surgeons, 35
percent of their incomes; internists, 29 percent; and radiologists,
28 percent.

Medicare is divided into Part A, Hospital Insurance, and Part B,
Supplementary Medical Insurance.

Part A is financed through payroll taxes and pays for inpatient
hospital care ($40 billion in 1984); stays in skilled nursing homes,
where a high degree of health care is provided ($550 million); and
home health ($1.8 billion) and hospice ($150 million) services.
Those sixty-five years old or older who are eligible for Social Security or Railroad Retirement are covered, as are the disabled. There
are deductibles, copayments, and limits on Medicare's hospital
and skilled nursing home benefits.* But Part A provides some hospice and home health care with no deductible or copayments. Reimbursement for hospice care particularly is designed to offer terminal patients an alternative to high-tech hospitalization.

Medicare's Part B, the Supplementary Medical Insurance Program, covers physicians' services in and out of the hospital, diagnostic tests, ambulance services, physical and speech therapy,
unlimited home health visits, and prosthetic devices and other
medical equipment. The beneficiary pays the first $75 of doctors'
bills; Medicare then pays 80 percent of the rest. Although participation in Part B is voluntary, 99 percent of the elderly and 92 percent of the disabled covered by Part A are enrolled. The monthly

---

* Medicare Part A pays in full for 60 days of inpatient hospital care for each
spell of illness, except for an up-front deductible based on the average national
cost of a hospital day ($400 in 1985). For the next 30 days, Medicare patients
must pay daily coinsurance equal to one-fourth the deductible. Medicare also
provides a lifetime reserve of 60 days. Part A also pays for stays in skilled nursing facilities for up to 100 days for each spell of illness. Beneficiaries must pay
coinsurance for each day over 20 equal to one-eighth the up-front hospital deductible.

premium ($16.60 in 1985), which is deducted from participants' Social Security checks, funds about 25 percent of Part B's $21 billion annual cost; the federal treasury bankrolls the rest.

Many medical services are not covered by Medicare: preventive measures (excepting pneumonia vaccines), outpatient drugs, eyeglasses, and basic dental services, for example. Medicare is decidedly tilted toward hospitalization. The rate of hospitalization of the elderly jumped 35 percent between 1970 and 1983.

Despite its limitations, Medicare has accomplished much of what it was designed to do. Virtually all the nation's elderly now have access to hospital care and substantial protection from the financial burden of hospitalization. Medicare was central to lowering death rates, which had held steady for twelve years, during the 1950s and early 1960s. Between 1968 and 1978, the number of deaths per 100,000 people decreased at an average annual rate of 1.5 percent for elderly men and 2.5 percent for elderly women. These declines were almost twice those Canada and Europe experienced over the same decade. Since the advent of Medicare (and Medicaid), life expectancy at age sixty-five has gone up two years; and since 1964 the two programs have helped stretch life expectancy at birth five years. In addition, the availability of procedures like cataract operations and hip and other joint surgery has much improved the quality of life for millions of elderly Americans.

On July 30, 1965, when President Johnson flew to Independence, Missouri, and signed the Medicare program into law with former President Harry Truman looking on, he gave older Americans a pep talk to join the program and then sent Secretary of Health, Education, and Welfare John Gardner, and all of us on the White House staff, hustling to get the elderly signed up for Medicare. It was a spectacularly successful effort. Just one year later, on July 1, 1966, Medicare opened its doors for business. During its first year, one in five of the elderly received hospital services under Medicare and some 70 percent of those enrolled in Part B received medical services. As its first year of operation ended, virtually all eligible elderly Americans were enrolled in Part A, Hospital Insurance, and 93 percent were enrolled in Part B, the voluntary Supplemental Medical Insurance Program.

But what price this glorious beginning?

Legislating no longer ends when the President signs into law a bill passed by Congress. That simply marks the time when the capital's street-smart turn their full attention to the executive branch and its rule makers. So it was with Medicare in 1965 and 1966. For the *i*'s and *t*'s the hospitals and doctors could not get Congress to dot and cross, they turned to the regulation-writers at the Department of Health, Education, and Welfare.

Under pressure from the medical industry, including threats that doctors and hospitals would not participate, and with the Johnson White House demanding a full-throttle program from day one, HEW gave away most of what was left in the store. While we were busy enrolling the elderly, we let the doctors and hospitals write reimbursement rules that would make them rich without any exposure to financial risk. In our zest to get Medicare off to a roaring start, we let them dig deep into the taxpayers' pockets.

Not only did doctors get from Congress the power to charge "reasonable," "customary," and "prevailing" fees, they also won, in the executive branch, significant control over how Medicare would set such fees.

The fee-for-service doctors mugged HMOs along the regulatory road. The statute Congress enacted was sufficiently broad, especially in the context of House and Senate committee reports, to allow alternative reimbursement procedures that would have strengthened health maintenance organizations and other prepaid group practice plans. But HEW's harassed administrators were so unwilling to nettle the medical establishment that HMOs were effectively foreclosed from participating in Medicare (and Medicaid).

The hospitals were even more persuasive with the HEW bureaucrats. They not only got interest on current and capital debt included in costs to be reimbursed, they also pressured HEW to agree to pay for depreciation on buildings and equipment they hadn't even bought themselves, buildings and equipment that had already been purchased with federal funds under the Hill-Burton Act. They got the depreciation on an accelerated (rather than a straight line) basis. The hospitals didn't even have to fund depreciation or set aside any prudent reserves. The for-profit hospitals and nursing homes got a minimum guarantee from the Congress in

1966: legislation to assure them a return on equity one and one-half times the return on government securities held by the Medicare hospital trust fund.

Just in case they left anything out, hospitals wanted a bonus from the taxpayers. HEW officials agreed to give them a 2 percent "plus factor" on top of their actual costs for treating Medicare patients. The 2 percent add-on was rationalized as compensating for a "lack of precision in cost funding in the early stages of program operation, as well as being in lieu of other elements of cost not specifically recognized." In fact, the 2 percent was a bribe to get the hospital industry to cooperate with Medicare. With this final windfall, the American Hospital Association promptly passed a resolution calling on all its members to support Medicare.

The price the doctors and hospitals exacted for Medicare's roaring start was fearsome. In the program's first year, the rate of increase in average daily hospital charges and physicians' fees doubled. In the summer of 1967, President Johnson asked HEW Secretary Gardner to identify "the reasons behind the rapid rise in the price of medical care and to offer recommendations for moderating that rise." Gardner reported that Medicare and its regulations were responsible for many price hikes. He was pessimistic but prescient when he told the President that in the future, the issue would not be "whether prices will rise, but how fast." The following year, in March 1968, when President Johnson sought legislative authority to use new methods of payment to stem rocketing costs, the Congress didn't have the stomach to take on the American Medical and Hospital associations.

Four years later, Medicare costs had jumped 60 percent, and Congress made the first of a series of legislative attempts to slow the rise. Instead of reimbursing hospitals for their daily patient costs, however rapidly they increased, Congress imposed payment caps on routine inpatient operating costs and established a system to slow construction of new hospital beds.

These 1972 amendments failed to moderate rising Medicare hospital costs. In 1974, the year the changes took effect, Medicare payments to hospitals jumped 30 percent (owing in part to the lifting of wage and price controls). They shot up another 25 percent in 1975, and 18 percent in both 1976 and 1977. Hospitals easily circumvented caps on rate increases by simply reclassifying "routine services" into "ancillary" services, which Medicare paid for separately, whatever the increase. Moreover, because intensive care units fell outside the routine service category, the legislation inadvertently encouraged hospitals to expand such expensive units and put more patients into them.

In addition to its effort to impose limits on hospital charges, in 1972 Congress created professional standards review organizations (PSROs), through which doctors reviewed their peers' work to ensure that services Medicare paid for were medically necessary, provided according to professional standards, and rendered at the appropriate level and length of stay of institutional care. The PSROs, by and large, lacked the gumption to take on their fellow physicians. Moreover, they did not have power to deny Medicare reimbursement to profligate providers. Thus, although a handful worked well, on the whole they did little to check the rise in doctors' fees or to trim the number, intensity, or length of hospital stays.

In 1974 Congress also sought to stop unnecessary hospital capital costs by financing health system agencies and states to review and approve health facility capital investments as a prerequisite to Medicare reimbursement. The health system agencies were unable to cope with local politics and every hospital's desire to have the latest CAT scanner or highest-tech intensive care unit. They were about as effective in slowing hospital construction as the old political postal department was in closing obsolete post offices. They were utterly ineffectual in eliminating excess hospital beds. Indeed, these agencies inadvertently created a perverse incentive: by establishing a cumbersome, often decidedly political regulatory apparatus that required a hospital to get a "certificate of need" before it could construct new beds, they encouraged hospitals to keep their old ones even when they didn't need them.

A BLANK CHECK FOR KIDNEY DIALYSIS

Prematurely predicting savings the 1972 amendments would achieve, Congress expanded Medicare coverage to some 1.7 million disabled persons under the age of sixty-five and to all under sixty-five suffering from end-stage renal disease (then some 18,000 people).

The end-stage renal disease program is a classic of effective lobbying by financially interested providers, human interest appeal, and generous-to-the-point-of-waste social policy. I can remember reviewing the 1967 budget with the Budget Director Charles Schultze and others in the Johnson administration, shortly before Christmas 1966. It had come to be widely recognized that kidney dialysis was effective and could make the difference between life and death for any American with end-stage renal disease. The law then provided such treatment—and hence life—for those eligible for veterans' benefits, for Medicare beneficiaries aged sixty-five and over, and for beneficiaries of Medicaid programs which covered this expensive procedure. There was a spirited, sometimes angry, discussion around the conference table in my White House West Wing office. Some said it was immoral not to provide care to all who needed it. Others said even the Great Society at its peak could not provide every medical service to all who needed it. But this was a matter of life itself, another heatedly added, pointing out that just because of quirks in the law, some were eligible and others not; some had the money to pay for it, others did not. The discussion went on and on.

We decided not to extend coverage for all kidney dialysis in the 1967 legislative program because we feared setting an expensive precedent and because of incipient concerns about becoming hostage to medical technology. But I tossed for several nights after making that decision and have thought about it many times since.

When Congress in 1972 legislated to provide kidney dialysis to all comers, the motivation was humane. But the costs have been staggering—not only because of the basic coverage, but also because Congress, bowing to the interests of hospitals and freestanding clinics, provided reimbursement for dialysis in these expensive settings, but not in the home.

Between 1972, when the law was passed, and 1977, the proportion of persons with end-stage renal disease receiving dialysis at home dropped from 40 percent to less than 10 percent. By 1977 the federal government was spending more than $1 billion each year to provide kidney dialysis for about 50,000 Americans, thousands of whom could have had dialysis in their own homes at savings of about 50 percent—hundreds of millions of dollars for taxpayers. When I discovered this, I urged Congress to reimburse patients for home dialysis as well. Fearing loss of big dollars, hospitals and clinic-based kidney dialysis businesses opposed my recommendations. After a lengthy struggle, their key congressional ally, Herman Talmadge, Democratic senator from Georgia, agreed to my proposal and the law was amended in 1978. Even so, in 1984 the federal government paid about $2 billion to provide dialysis to 78,000 Americans.

CAPPING HOSPITAL CHARGES

In April 1977, I recommended that the Congress limit all hospital charges to a rate of increase one and one-half times that of the consumer price index, a reduction from the two-and-a-half-times pace then prevalent. We sought the lid as a temporary measure while we plotted fundamental changes in the reimbursement system. The potential savings from our legislation was $53 billion in the first five years.

In March 1979, in response to hospital industry concerns, we modified our proposal, suggesting a cap based on the cost of the market basket of goods and services hospitals purchased, plus 1 percent. But effective and well-bankrolled lobbying by profit-making hospitals, the American Hospital and Medical associations, and the medical equipment manufacturers, a powerful anti-regulatory sentiment in the Congress, and our inability to get the American people to appreciate the financial significance to them of hospital-cost containment killed the bill. While our legislation was pending in 1978 and 1979, Medicare payments to hospitals increased at an average annual rate of just over 14 percent, a drop from the 18.2 percent rate of increase in 1977. But once the industry killed the legislation, Medicare hospital costs jumped 22.4 percent in 1980 and 20.6 percent in 1981.

In 1980 and 1981 Congress chipped away at the health care cost problem for which it bore so much responsibility. In 1980 it passed an assortment of measures designed to moderate Medicare (and Medicaid) cost increases, principally by authorizing full rather than partial payment for less expensive care, such as certain surgical procedures performed in a physician's office or an outpatient center, and home health services. This legislation also supported state programs regulating hospital rates; restricted access to Medicare (and Medicaid) by providers found to have defrauded programs or patients; put nonphysicians on professional standards review organizations; and limited Medicare payments in accident cases to reimbursement, if any was still warranted, after the insurance company, no fault insurance, or person at fault had first paid.

In 1981 Congress tried more quick fixes to control Medicare costs. It increased the patient deductible under both Parts A and B, stepped up reimbursement of home health agencies, required that private health insurance held by kidney dialysis patients cover the first year of treatment, and further stiffened fraud penalties. In a rare action to change the health care system rather than merely shift its burdens, Congress authorized federal reimbursement of costs of eliminating excess hospital beds or converting them to nursing home use.

But tinkering did not do the job. Though inflation in the overall economy cooled, health care costs continued to boil. In the last three months of 1981, the consumer price index increased at an annual rate of only 3 percent, while the index for hospital rooms rocketed up at a rate of 20 percent and doctors' fees at 10.6 percent. Senator Robert Dole, who had opposed earlier cost-containment legislation, suggested in March 1982 that Congress might have made a mistake by not adopting the proposals I had made earlier.

In 1982 Congress put new caps on routine inpatient operating costs Medicare would pay for and, having once been burned, capped costs of intensive care units and ancillary services like laboratories as well. The 1982 law limited the annual rate of increase in operating expenses per case to the rise in the hospital wage and price index plus 1 percent. (This was essentially the lid I had proposed as HEW Secretary, but Congress limited its application to Medicare.) For the first time, hospitals whose costs increased less than the limit could keep part of the difference; those whose costs exceeded the limit would get just one-fourth of the additional costs for no more than two years. Congress also wiped out a nursing differential that Medicare had paid to cover what hospitals claimed were higher costs of caring for Medicare patients. (Hospitals had been given this bounty when, in 1969, the overall 2 percent plus factor was eliminated from Medicare reimbursement.)

To increase revenues, Congress applied Medicare to federal employees, required them to pay the 1.3 percent payroll tax, and again upped the premium for Medicare Part B beneficiaries.* To foster competitive systems, Congress authorized prospective payments to HMOs enrolling Medicare beneficiaries and reimbursement for hospice services. Congress also closed down the PSRO program, in which physicians attempted to police themselves, and instead directed Medicare to contract directly with peer review organizations (PROs), which were given the power to withhold reimbursement in cases of inappropriate care.

Senate Finance Committee Chairman Dole's sleeper in the 1982 law was the requirement that the Health and Human Services Department submit to Congress, within five months, a new prospective payment system for hospitals and nursing homes. The report was submitted in December 1982. Hospitals, faced with increasing legislative restrictions under the old system, found prospective payment the lesser of the evils they confronted. Against estimates that Medicare faced bankruptcy by 1987, Congress acted swiftly, and on April 20, 1983, President Reagan signed into law authorization for the sweeping new system establishing 470 diagnosis related groups with per-case charges for specific medical conditions set in advance, regardless of the actual costs incurred by hospitals. Payments to for-profit hospitals of a net return on equity continued at a reduced rate, and cost-based reimbursement for hospital capital facilities and equipment remained. But the law contemplates folding them into the DRG payments after a temporary reprieve.

* Since 1974, the portion of Part B costs these premiums covered had dropped from 47 to 24 percent. In 1982 Congress required that such premiums cover 25 percent of Part B costs.

FREEZING PHYSICIANS' FEES

Congressional attempts to stem the rise in Medicare payments to physicians have been frustrating. After a beneficiary pays the $75 deductible, Medicare picks up 80 percent of what it determines to be reasonable charges for physicians' services. Until 1976, Congress calculated such charges each year on the basis of what the physician and similar physicians in the area had charged the year before. This allowed doctors to step up the level of Medicare reimbursement by increasing their own fees. In 1976 Congress set up a Medicare Economic Index that limited the annual rate of increase in physicians' fees to the rate of increase in their costs. So from 1976 to 1983 Medicare physicians' fees were calculated by multiplying the 1973 fees by the current index. But since physicians had no incentive to be cost-conscious, and since the index was designed to maintain their rate of return on costs, payments to physicians continued to rise at annual rates averaging 19 percent from 1976 to 1983.

Moreover, doctors need not accept Medicare's determination of the reasonable fee as payment in full; they may charge whatever they can get from patients. Until 1984, up to 30 percent of doctors always charged more than Medicare's reasonable fee and another 50 percent frequently did so. Only 18 percent of physicians treating Medicare patients always accepted the program's reasonable fee as full payment. The additional charge rose sharply: from an average of 13.6 percent of the reasonable fee in the mid-1970s to nearly 25 percent in the early 1980s. In 1983, 80 percent of physicians' bills to Medicare exceeded the program's allowable fees by a total of $5.6 billion.

In 1983 Part B of Medicare, which pays the doctors' bills, spent almost $20 billion, a sum that was projected to more than double by 1989, to $43 billion. Facing these projections, Congress in July 1984 slapped a fifteen-month freeze on physicians' fees Medicare would pay.* Doctors were still not required to accept Medicare's reasonable fee as payment in full, but those who did have been

---

* The same legislation set a fee schedule for payments to independent laboratories for test performed on Medicare patients.

promised an advantage in calculating new fees after the freeze. Congress also created a program to speed checks to physicians who accept Medicare's reasonable fee as full payment and to publicize their acceptance to the elderly. The initial response has increased from 18 to 30 percent the share of physicians who accept Medicare's reasonable fee in all cases.

The changes in the hospital reimbursement, the freeze in doctors' fees, and the general decline in overall inflation seem to have deferred the day of reckoning for Medicare. But the continuing importance of workable cost containment can be gleaned not only from Medicare's near-term bankruptcy problems, but from projections that if the program remains unchanged, its outlays will have to be reduced by 19 percent, or payroll taxes will have to be increased by 24 percent, over the next twenty-five years.

MEDICAID

Created in 1965 along with Medicare, Medicaid is quite different in terms of financing, administration, and people served.

Medicare is very much an insurance program for the elderly and disabled, regardless of income. It is entirely a federal government enterprise, financed through payroll taxes, premiums paid by those covered, and general tax revenues. Medicaid is essentially a grant program, jointly funded by the federal and state governments. While the federal government pays just over 50 percent of the Medicaid bill, its share varies state by state, from 50 to 78 percent, depending on per capita income, the proportion of Medicaid recipients in each state, and other factors.

Medicaid covers about 22 million Americans, primarily those poor people who qualify for the two big welfare programs: Aid to Families with Dependent Children (AFDC), which covers 5 million parents (almost 90 percent single-parent women) and 9 million children, and Supplemental Security Income (SSI), which covers 6 million aged, blind, and disabled people. States largely determine whom Medicaid will cover, because they set many standards for welfare eligibility. Moreover, federal law permits states to provide Medicaid assistance to the "medically needy"—

individuals whose incomes are too high to enable them to qualify for AFDC or SSI, but too low to cover their medical bills.

Federal law requires states to provide a minimum level of services to Medicaid recipients: inpatient and outpatient hospital care; laboratory and X-ray services; skilled nursing-home care and home health services for those twenty-one and older; examination and treatment for children under twenty-one; family planning and rural health clinics. About half of Medicaid spending goes for federally mandated services. States have the discretion to provide additional coverage. States pay health care providers directly for services to patients and almost invariably require physicians to accept the state fees as full payment.

AFDC children and parents are about 70 percent of Medicaid recipients, but they receive less than 30 percent of the program's funds. The aged, blind, disabled, and others make up the remaining 30 percent of the recipients, and they receive more than 70 percent of all Medicaid spending. Medicaid spends 43 cents of every dollar on nursing-home care for 7 percent of its beneficiaries, 30 cents on inpatient hospital care, 21 cents on outpatient and physician services, and 6 cents on ancillary services like lab tests, X-rays, and prescription drugs. Though they are only 10 percent of the institutionalized Medicaid population, the mentally retarded receive 28 percent of the dollars spent for institutional care.

Medicaid, saddled with the same cost-based, fee-for-service payment system for hospitals and doctors as Medicare, has also been plagued by relentlessly rising costs. From combined federal and state payments of $4 billion in 1968, Medicaid has grown to $39 billion in 1984. Between 1972 and 1981, Medicaid payments rose at an annual rate of 17 percent, driving many state budgets into deficit and imposing increased demands for revenues. Medicaid's share of our nation's health bill has been between 10 and 11 percent since 1980.

Since the mid-1970s, Congress and the states have tried to slow rising costs. Since 1980 Congress has held down the federal share and provided states with flexibility and incentives to control costs. In 1981 federal legislation reduced the amount of federal Medicaid payments to the states by an increasing percentage in each of the next three years, up to a 4.5 percent reduction in 1984. Each state could trim the amount of the federal cut: by 1 percent if it had a qualified cost-review program; by another 1 percent if its unemployment rate was 150 percent or more of the national average; and by an additional 1 percent if its recoveries from fraud and abuse equaled 1 percent of its federal payment. Other congressional changes sought to eliminate unnecessary hospitalization and encourage day care for the elderly at home or in the community rather than in nursing homes.

In 1980 and 1981 federal lawmakers also encouraged states to move from "reasonable cost" reimbursement of hospitals, nursing homes, and other providers to a more stringent standard: costs reasonable and adequate for efficient and economically operated facilities. In addition, Congress allowed states to pay family doctors to guide patients through the health care system, to share savings with prudent patients who sought less costly care, such as HMOs, and to require recipients to get nonemergency treatment from cost-effective providers only, in order to stop unnecessary use of expensive hospital emergency rooms.

By 1984, twenty-four states had moved to make many of the changes, and twenty-three had at least some Medicaid enrollees in prepaid plans, like HMOs. California created a czar to contract with lowest bidders to provide Medicaid services and saved $165 million in the first year of its new program. Illinois and Nebraska also adopted systems for competitive contracting with hospitals. In 1985 ten states had shifted to their own DRG systems for reimbursing Medicaid hospital care; four other states were moving in that direction. Most states are tightening up on their payments to nursing homes—so much so that many operators fear they will not be able to meet their costs.

Since 1982 Congress has permitted the states to impose copayments on patients for mandatory as well as discretionary benefits and has further tightened eligibility and reduced benefits. The service most frequently targeted for copayment (nineteen states) is prescription drugs. Alabama, Idaho, and Kentucky have reduced the number of hospital days they will cover. Several states have also restricted the drugs and number of physician visits covered. By 1984, the annual increase in Medicaid expenditures had slowed to just over 7 percent.

Medicaid has been a major force in improving the health of millions of Americans. Between 1970 and 1978 adult death rates dropped more than twice as fast as they did between 1959 and 1967, in good measure because the poor were given access to health care. Between 1968 and 1980 deaths from illnesses that hit the poor hardest went down sharply: 53 percent for influenza and pneumonia; 52 percent for tuberculosis; 31 percent for diabetes. Adult deaths during childbirth dropped 72 percent. Since 1964 life expectancy for black females has jumped from 66 to 73 years. By 1984, for the first time in our history, a black baby girl had a life expectancy greater than a white baby boy. Infant mortality was cut from 25 deaths per 1,000 in 1964 to 10.6 per 1,000 twenty years later. The disparity for black infants persists, but even among blacks, infant mortality dropped from 42 per 1,000 to less than 20 per 1,000 over the same period.

Cuts since 1981 in Medicaid and related health programs underscore the importance of those programs to the poor. The rate of decline in infant mortality slowed to 2.7 percent in 1983, down from an annual average of 4.6 percent from 1965 to 1982. As the feds reduced spending on immunization programs, the incidence of measles rose in 1984 for the first time since the vaccine was introduced in 1963. Hypertension patients dropped from Medicaid experience an average rise in blood pressure that increases their risk of fatal heart attack by 40 percent.

Among the poor there is still an enormous unmet need for health care in America. In 1985, the Department of Health and Human Services found that minorities suffer 60,000 unnecessary deaths each year, largely from heart and respiratory disease, stroke, cancer, and infant mortality rates higher than those among whites. In 1984, even though some states broadened eligibility as their economies improved, less than half of Americans in poverty received Medicaid. Since 1977, as eligibility for welfare has been curbed, the proportion of the poor covered by Medicaid has declined. The number of people in poverty has grown by more than 10 million, while the number receiving Medicaid has dropped by more than 1 million. The health care needs of our nation's poor will be too expensive to meet without a restructured delivery system.

FRAUD, ABUSE, AND WASTE

The federal government and the states have been moving to deal with the demons of fraud, abuse, and waste in Medicaid and Medicare. It's far easier to do with Medicare, which is a single program, operated by the federal government through companies that process claims for payment, with individual eligibility easy to determine: those over sixty-five and those receiving Social Security disability payments.

Medicaid is a much tougher nut to crack. It's not one program but more than fifty different health plans—one for each state, the District of Columbia, and the territories. Each jurisdiction sets its own income level for determining eligible individuals or families. Each has wide discretion to establish which health care services to cover and what to pay providers. The millions of Medicaid transactions that occur in this complex administrative maze are prone to error, fraud, and abuse. Much of the waste is a result of Medicaid's inherent complexity. Determinations of eligibility turn on such fine points that it is not possible to train thousands of individuals to administer the program with accuracy, even in the age of miracle computers. Most leakage of Medicaid funds stems from errors by state and local administrators struggling with infernally complex and hydra-headed programs.

As Secretary of HEW, I pressed hard to get states to set up fraud and abuse units, and Congress provided funds to get them started. By 1984 thirty-four states had Medicaid fraud-control units, which each year prosecute hundreds of offenders and collect millions of dollars in fines, overpayments, and restitutions. Congress is requiring states to clean up their Medicaid programs or pay penalties.

Until Medicaid is simplified, however, fraud and abuse will remain difficult to control. The potential scams are endless. In one case, a storefront health clinic and nearby shoe store charged Medicaid for orthopedic shoes, while providing patients with low-quality everyday footwear. In August 1984, after a two-month investigation, the *New York Daily News* revealed that newspaper reporters armed with Medicaid cards got drugs of high street value, such as Valium, Elavil, Librium, and codeine, virtually on request, after less than ten minutes of examination, from physicians specializing in Medicaid patients. Junkies frequently obtain prescription drugs this way, then sell them to support their habits.

THE VETERANS

Medicare, with a big assist from Medicaid, may set the pace for health care delivery and reimbursement. But looming behind is a health care system with costs simmering like a volcano preparing to erupt: the Veterans Administration.

As the number of veterans sixty-five and over grows—from some 4 million in 1984 to 7.2 million in 1990 and close to 10 million in 2000—so will the demands on the VA's system of health care for the nation's vets. Unchecked, that health care bill could go from $9 billion in 1984 (60 percent for hospital care) to $50 billion in 2000.

Conceived and born in an age when we fought wars to end all wars, when no expense was too much for returning vets, when life expectancy was barely over sixty-five, when there was no Medicare or Medicaid, and when we hadn't invented multimillion-dollar machines to keep us breathing a few more days, the VA health care system has used the flag to protect itself from any serious cost-containment efforts. Lyndon Johnson's attempts to close VA hospitals in the wake of Medicare sputtered. President Carter rejected out of hand my suggestion that veterans' hospitals be included in the cost-containment cap we proposed to Congress.

In 1984 the VA operated 172 medical centers and hospitals with 80,000 beds, 226 outpatient clinics, 101 nursing homes with 9,000 beds, 16 veterans' homes, plus a variety of programs for home care and geriatric day and residential care. It employed about 200,000 medical workers of its own and contracted for health care services from other providers and specialists. The VA's medical centers provide care to some 1.3 million inpatients each year and accommodate nearly 17 million outpatient visits. The VA finances about 25 million inpatient days of hospital care and some 9 million inpatient days in nursing homes. It also pays for some 2 million visits to non-VA physicians each year.

Access to care is governed through a system of priorities, with veterans who need treatment for service-connected injuries or illnesses at the top. But as a practical matter, if a veteran needs hospital care, he gets it, whatever his priority on paper. By 1984, 70 percent of the VA's hospital patients and 67 percent of its nursing-home patients had no service-connected disabilities.

The Congressional Budget Office estimates that by 1990 expenses for the medical care system the VA operates will jump to $15.4 billion. Assuming that the VA continues to serve veterans in the same kinds of VA facilities as it used in 1984, between 1985 and 1990 it will have to spend $400 million for new nursing homes and $3 billion to renovate and replace hospital facilities. By the year 2000, unless current usage patterns change, the Congressional Budget Office thinks the VA will need another 29,000 hospital beds and 40,000 nursing-home beds. The VA considers these numbers too conservative; it seeks to add as many as 108,000 new hospital beds and at least 102,000 nursing home beds by the year 2000.

If there is no change in the law or our health care delivery systems, the estimate of the VA is far closer to the real world year 2000 than that of the Congressional Budget Office. Why? By the year 2000, owing to the surge of aging World War II, Korean War, and Vietnam War veterans and their increased longevity, the number of veterans sixty-five and over—all of whom are eligible for free care—will more than double, approaching 10 million. In 1984 there were more than 200,000 veterans eighty-five and older; by the year 2000, there will be more than 300,000. Elderly veterans represented 10.6 of all veterans in 1980; by 2000 their share will approach 40 percent, and (barring a major war) remain at that level for another 30 years.

Unlike Medicare, the VA charges no premiums, copayments, or deductibles. As one elderly veteran at a VA hospital in Hines, Illinois, put it when he learned he might need coronary bypass surgery: under Medicare, his piece of the $20,000 bill would have been $3,000 to $4,000; under the VA, it was zero.

THE ARMY, NAVY, AIR FORCE, MARINES—AND AMERICAN INDIANS

At a cost around $9 billion, the Department of Defense runs its own health care system for members and retirees of the armed forces and their dependents and survivors, some 10 million people, including 2 million men and women on active duty. The Department operates 165 hospitals as well as hundreds of clinics. Its hospitals provide some 5.5 million inpatient days of care each year.

DOD also finances 2.5 million days of inpatient care outside its facilities through the Civilian Health and Medical Program of the Uniformed Services (CHAMPUS), mainly for dependents of active personnel and for retirees, who use civilian hospitals when military facilities are not available to them.

The Indian Health Service, yet another federal health care delivery system, provides health care and public health services to some 885,000 Indians and Alaskan natives through a network of hospitals and clinics. In 1984 this system cost some $500 million.

STATE AND LOCAL GOVERNMENT: THE NOT SO LITTLE NEPHEWS AND NIECES

In 1984, America's fifty states and 50,000 cities, counties, and towns paid some $50 billion for health care. They spent $32 billion to run hospitals, neighborhood clinics, and school health programs, to treat alcoholics and drug addicts, to institutionalize the mentally ill, and for a host of public health efforts. In addition, they put up approximately $18 billion just to pay their share of the Medicaid bill.

Hospitals and physicians took the largest portion of the money that states and localities spent on health care. The next largest slice, about $10 billion, went to pay for state and local public health efforts, for activities ranging from fighting flu epidemics to reducing teenage pregnancy. States, mostly the larger ones like New York and California, and cities spent $2 billion to pay for medical care for poor people not covered by Medicaid. Localities, and to a far lesser extent states, financed some 1,715 acute-care hospitals and 56 psychiatric and other specialty hospitals.

For state and local governments, as for their big federal uncle, health care costs loom as a foreboding financial cloud on the budgetary horizon.

Chapter 9

THE GREAT HEALTH CARE COST SHELL GAME

In an economic system based on a truly free market, competition itself delivers the best product at the lowest cost. When one supplier lowers his price to a customer, other suppliers follow suit or lose the business. Suppliers compete with each other for buyers, who drive hard bargains because in turn they face stiff competition. So a supplier can't jack up costs to one buyer in order to recoup revenues lost because he sold to another at a lower price.

That's not the way the health care system has worked. Because health care suppliers have not delivered in a competitive environment and the patient-buyers are not competing with each other, hospitals and doctors have been able to shift costs and charges from one patient to another.

In such a system, attempts to control costs can easily turn into a shell game. This has been particularly true for the federal government. Since the late 1970s, the federal government has sought aggressively to cap the amount it will pay to treat beneficiaries of programs like Medicare. Unfortunately, the structure of the health care industry is such that these caps produce largely illusory savings as long as the suppliers can shift costs to other purchasers or other parts of the system.

Congress puts a cap on Medicare payments to hospitals, and the hospitals move the cost to the states and other customers. States put their own caps on Medicaid hospital payments, and the hospitals slip the pea to the private insurers and the Blues.

Congress establishes caps on medical procedures in hospitals and the doctors move the pea outside the hospital to their offices or clinics. As a result, the House Select Committee on Aging reported, there has been a huge increase in cataract surgery outside the hospital, with doctors in 1985 billing $1.2 billion above what Medicare pays under the DRG system for the same operation. And sales of diagnostic equipment to doctors and laboratories, to enable them to perform in their offices or labs tests once done in hospitals, have rocketed, with predictions they will soar from less than $200 million in 1984 to more than $1 billion by the end of the decade. So the government, running around like a Looney-Tunes cat pawing for a mouse under a blanket, rushes to set a fee schedule for payments to independent laboratories for outpatient tests performed on Medicare patients.

Medicare's diagnosis related groups are a step in the right direction. But even this DRG system is part of the Great Health Care Cost Shell Game. It lets the hospitals shift the pea to the states and private insurers, and to settings outside their doors.

Sleight-of-hand tricks do not reduce health care costs. Costs disappearing from the federal health care budget have a remarkable ability to reappear elsewhere in the system. In the case of many elderly patients, for example, the incentive in the Medicare DRG cap for early discharge of hospital patients translates into early admission to nursing homes. The federal government plays this shell game because Medicaid and individuals pay for most nursing-home care, and the states pay half the Medicaid bill. In contrast, the federal government gets no state help in paying the Medicare bill.

Pressure to get the elderly from hospital to nursing home is not the only shell game the feds play with the states. In 1982 Congress cut the federal Medicaid contribution by 3 percent for a $400 million reduction in federal spending. But there were no savings to our society. These costs were shifted to the states, which in turn raised costs to recipients by reducing benefits or eliminating Medicaid eligibility. The Urban Institute found that the 1981–1982 recession would have added more than 1 million people to Medicaid if government "cost savings" had not produced an actual decrease of 1.2 million Medicaid recipients. As a result, hundreds of thousands of poor persons either assumed the cost of expensive medical care, did without, or (if they were lucky) became charity cases at hospitals and emergency rooms, many of which increased charges to the privately well-insured to compensate for lost revenues. But none of these changes helped make the health delivery system more efficient.

Another variant of the health care cost shell game is the trend to ambulatory surgery, which has spurred enormous new investments in equipment and physical plant for outpatient surgery centers, without any concomitant reduction in the number of hospital beds. As a result, most hospitals have even more empty and unnecessary beds than formerly, and the same high fixed costs must now be spread over fewer patients. Unfortunately, when caps of one kind or another provide incentives to act more efficiently, we do not get the full benefit of the savings. Unless we require hospitals to close down or convert to other uses beds no longer needed because of the move to less expensive outpatient surgery and preadmission testing, they will simply shift the pea of higher costs under the shells of fewer patients.

Too often, government changes in Medicare and Medicaid have been piecemeal and have not eliminated inefficiencies and waste in the system. The federal government and the states have been quick to grab credit for reducing budget deficits, when in fact they are only hiding health care costs under another shell. Rather than attack the structural defects in the health care financing system, the Congress has usually opted to impose a hidden tax on American citizens and American business. The federal government's "savings" are increased costs for business and individuals.

Under Medicare, for example, the federal government has shifted costs to individuals as well as to private payers like Chrysler. The vast majority of our elderly citizens are not independently wealthy or covered by generous retirement health benefits. For them, the savings the government achieves through increases in Medicare deductibles, premiums, and copayments and reductions in benefits translate into financial hardship. Between 1982 and 1984, the Medicare Part B premium, covering physicians' services and outpatient care, went from $115 to $200 per year. For many, the government's cost savings have increased out-of-pocket premium costs by 75 percent.

In 1966 a Medicare beneficiary had to pay the first $40 of each hospital stay; in 1985 that initial payment hit $400. Over the same time, the daily copayment a Medicare beneficiary is required to make for long-term hospital stays (for the sixtieth to the ninetieth day after admission) has jumped from $10 to $100 per day. Our citizens haven't saved anything. Our government has simply hidden the pea under another shell.

In 1984 elderly Medicare beneficiaries paid an estimated average of $1,600 to $1,700 for medical services not covered by Medicare, including rising Medicare deductibles and copayments. This represents 15 to 16 percent of the 1984 estimated average annual income ($10,615) of Americans sixty-five and older. For some two-thirds of elderly Medicare beneficiaries, out-of-pocket spending includes premiums for private "Medigap" insurance policies, which pay for Medicare deductibles and copayments and, increasingly, to replace reduced benefits. In 1984 premiums for Medigap policies ranged from $300 to $500 per year, with comprehensive policies costing $1,000 or more. Again, the pea keeps moving to another shell, with no structural change in the system.

Not all deductibles and copayments are shell game variants. They can give the individual employee a sense that health care is not a free lunch. As my Chrysler experiences demonstrate, the imposition of copayments and deductibles on expensive and inefficient fee-for-service physician and cost-based hospital plans can furnish an economic incentive for employees to shift to more efficient health care systems, like preferred providers and health maintenance organizations for which no copayment or deductible is imposed. Focused copayments and deductibles can be employed to encourage patients to seek care is less expensive settings—for example, to use home health care services in lieu of entering a nursing home, or to receive tests in a physician's office rather than in a hospital. Under these circumstances, copayments and deductibles can help effect structural changes in the health care system. Still, their use is hard to justify in the case of the old and the poor and cannot alone effect structural changes.

Look at what government "cost savings" have meant to American businesses.

From 1983 to 1984, medical costs for many corporations jumped 20 to 25 percent, as Medicare's DRG system capped federal payments to hospitals. In the noncompetitive health care system, hospitals could make up for reduced Medicare payments and declining occupancy by raising rates to private payers. Deere & Co. stated that it had actually reduced hospital use by its employees, "but higher costs wiped out the savings," as hospitals shifted to private payers charges Medicare would no longer pay.

In 1984 Chrysler paid for health care for nearly as many retirees and dependents as active employees and their dependents. For its retirees, Chrysler, like other American corporations, pays for many health care services for which Medicare does not pick up the bill. Therefore, as Medicare seeks to ease its own financial crisis by shifting costs to the individual, if that beneficiary is a Chrysler retiree, Chrysler picks up the tab. The 1985 increases in the hospital deductible alone cost Chrysler more than $1 million a year.

The Tax Equity and Fiscal Responsibility Act of 1982 (TEFRA) requires employers to offer employees sixty-five to sixty-nine years old and their dependents the same health insurance coverage that they provide other employees. For employees in this age group who choose their employer's plan, Medicare becomes the secondary rather than the primary coverage. That provision does not save Americans a single dollar. It simply shifts the pea from Medicare to the private sector. The cost to Chrysler was $1.4 million in 1983 and increases annually. The cost to all U.S. businesses was more than $1.5 billion in 1983.

Some proposals for rescuing Medicare are outrageous examples of the Great Health Care Cost Shell Game. The Advisory Council on Social Security proposal to delay Medicare eligibility from age sixty-five to age sixty-seven would cost Chrysler approximately $100 million over five years. Over ten years, the delay would cost American business and citizens some $75 billion. It would shift the cost directly to those citizens not fortunate enough to have coverage through retirement plans. And it would not eliminate a single dollar of waste or inefficiency in the health care system.

The states play the Great Health Care Cost Shell Game with Chrysler and American businesses as well. In Michigan, Blue Cross was allowed to shift $2 million in bad debts to Chrysler bills in 1984. Medicare and Medicaid do not permit hospitals to shift bad debts to them. The Michigan State Insurance Commissioner directed the Blues to charge private payers to help subsidize the costs of insurance to supplement Medicare coverage of senior citizens.

The pea that gets shifted from the public sector shell to the private sector shell is so large that it's hard to hide.

The Health Insurance Association of America, representing the commercial insurers, estimates that cost shifting to private payers jumped from $5.8 billion in 1982 to $8.8 billion in 1984. The association's testimony before the Joint Economic Committee of the Congress was blunt:

> ... hospitals recoup reductions in Medicare and Medicaid reimbursement by inflating charges to private patients. Those who are insured face higher premiums. Those who are not—such as laid-off workers who have lost their insurance—are faced with a ruinous hidden tax exacted at a time when they are least able to pay—a tax on their already sky-rocketing hospital charges.

Indigent care at hospitals, both public and private, is another constantly moving pea in the cruelest health care shell game. Most often, hospitals have simply folded the cost of uncompensated care, whether rendered voluntarily or in the form of bad debts, into their overall costs and then passed it along to private payers—individuals, commercial insurers, and the Blues. For years, it was generally accepted that the affluent and well-insured could be charged more in order to pay for health care for the poor. Medicare is prohibited by law from paying for these expenses, since they represent services provided to non-Medicare patients.

By 1984 the total cost of charity care at American hospitals approached $8 billion. When the costs of indigent care become too great for a hospital to shift them to other payers, the ultimate in cost shifting, "patient dumping," takes place. Private hospitals—both nonprofit and profit-making—simply refuse to admit most uninsured poor patients; those they have to accept because their condition is life-threatening are transferred to public hospitals as fast as possible. The CBS News broadcast *60 Minutes* recorded these words of a doctor at Dallas–Fort Worth Medical Center, a private hospital, who called Parkland, a public hospital, seeking to transfer a patient: "Listen to me for a minute now, don't give me all that crap. She does not have any insurance. The hospital [Dallas–Fort Worth] does not want to take care of her, OK.... This is a private capitalistic money-making hospital. They're on my back to have her transferred."

In 1984 Cook County Hospital in Chicago admitted 6,000 emergency patients transferred from other facilities, up five times since 1981. In Washington, D.C., the number of patients transferred for financial reasons from private nonprofit hospitals to the city's public hospital, D.C. General, increased more than five times between 1981 and 1984, from 169 to 904. The president of one of D.C.'s nonprofit hospitals claimed that the transfers were necessary because the proportion of free care provided by his hospital had increased from 8 to 11 percent. The executive vice president of American Medical International, a for-profit hospital chain, put it this way: "We don't expect Safeway or A&P to give away free food for people who can't afford it."

This cruel shifting simply dumps the health care problem on public hospitals, further jeopardizing their already precarious position, and it often endangers the life and health of the patient moved.

It's time to stop playing shell games.

True reductions in costs will come only from fundamental changes in the way we deliver and pay for health care. Those changes require action by all the players: employers and unions, the administration and the Congress, federal, state, and local governments, lawyers, and the doctors, hospitals, laboratories, drug companies, and other suppliers—and patients.

Government in particular has got to get its act together, stop playing the health care cost shell game, and turn its attention to instituting some system-wide reforms.

Federal, state, and local governments pay more than 50 percent of the costs of hospital care and 30 percent of the doctors' bills. When Medicare moves to a DRG system, private payers and states must act quickly or suffer shifted costs. California recognized this when it started soliciting lowest bidders to provide Medicaid services. At the same time, seeing the potential for up to $800 million of cost shifting to private payers, the California legislature authorized private insurance companies and Blue Cross to contract with selected providers and lowest bidders, and to require policyholders to use their services. Massachusetts set up a statewide prospective payment program that fixes hospital budgets and attempts to defeat cost shifting by freezing payment levels for all payers. By 1984 ten states claimed comprehensive cost-containment systems, and more than 800 cost-containment bills were before the legislatures of the fifty states, most of those bills prone to cost shifting. But unless federal and state cost-containment measures focus on the difference between playing a shell game and changing the system, the good efforts springing up across America from corporations, unions, commercial insurers, the Blues, and many doctors and hospitals will sputter, and the true potential of America's health care revolution will be lost.

There isn't much time left to get an efficient health care delivery system. The graying of America is forcing the issue, with a rapidly increasing number of older citizens demanding more and more care in expensive high-technology hospitals and nursing homes. Our nation cannot tolerate the shell game much longer.

Chapter 10

OF NURSING HOMES, GOLDEN PONDS, AND DEATH CONTROL

Perhaps no more severe test of compassion and morality lies ahead for the American nation and its people than how we confront the crisis of our exploding elderly population. Nothing brings that crisis into sharper relief than the needs we face for long-term care.

Consider nursing homes, perhaps the most visible manifestation of the crisis.

Despite swindles in New York State and elsewhere, persisting tales of exploitation and charges of drugging the vulnerable elderly with tranquilizers, since 1965 nursing homes have been the fastest-growing sector of the health care industry—and they still haven't been able to keep up with demand.

In 1960 Americans spent $500 million on nursing homes, less than 2 percent of the money they put up for personal health care. In 1984 Americans spent $32 billion, almost 10 percent of what they paid for personal health care—and 70 percent of the people who need long-term care aren't even in nursing homes! In 1990 Americans will spend about $60 billion on nursing homes, just about double what they spent in 1984.

The two biggest social reasons for this increase in nursing-home care are the aging of our citizens and the mobility of Americans. The increase in the number of older citizens by itself requires new nursing homes. On top of that, more and more Americans live and work hundreds of miles from their parents. Senior citizens—those who can—often retire to the warm climates of Florida and Arizona, leaving their working children far behind in the Northeast or Midwest.

But need alone is insufficient to support a massive expansion of social services. Money is the other key ingredient. Here, to a degree few appreciate, the Great Society's Medicaid program created a major industry. Most Americans think of Medicaid as a program to pay poor people's hospital and doctors' bills. Actually, Medicaid bankrolls half of all nursing home outlays. Medicaid has been the driving force in the startling growth of nursing homes for the mentally retarded: in the ten years since 1974, when Congress authorized payment for such institutionalized care, spending has shot from $203 million to more than $4 billion a year. Medicare, Veterans Administration, and other federal, state, and local payments bring the government's share of the nursing-home bill to 54 percent. Private insurance pays less than 2 percent. The remaining 44 percent of nursing-home bills are directly paid by individual residents and their relatives, especially their children. But government is getting increasingly reluctant to pick up any more of the tab. Future costs are so astronomical that when in 1978, as Secretary of HEW, I was putting together a national health plan, my first decision was not to cover long-term care.

The nursing-home industry differs from the hospital business. Despite the rise in for-profit chains, hospitals are predominantly nonprofit in structure. In sharp contrast, 70 percent of the 1.5 million nursing-home beds are in institutions owned and operated for profit. About 340,000 beds are in homes, often with a religious affiliation, run on a not-for-profit basis. State and local governments maintain the other 125,000 beds. There are lots more nursing homes than hospitals—23,000 as opposed to fewer than 7,000 hospitals—and they're smaller. The average hospital stay is less than ten days; the median (i.e., most frequent) nursing-home stay is 79 days, but because some patients (the mentally and physically disabled as well as the elderly) remain in nursing homes for long periods, the average stay overall is 456 days. One survey concluded that 16 percent of nursing-home residents have been there five years or more; 15 percent, from three to five years; and 33 percent from one to three years. Hospitals have scores of thousands of excess beds. Nursing-home occupancy rates approach 95 percent, and most have long waiting lists.

While the supply of available nursing-home beds has grown steadily, it has not kept pace with the increasing numbers of the oldest of the elderly. Over the ten years from 1975 to 1984, the ranks of the elderly eighty-five and up increased at an average annual rate of 4 percent, while the number of nursing-home beds grew at a rate of less than 3 percent. These very elderly people are fifteen times more likely to be institutionalized than those sixty-five to seventy-four. Roughly 22 percent of those over eighty-five are in nursing homes, compared with 7 percent of those between seventy-five and eighty-four, and 1.5 percent of those sixty-five to seventy-four.

Precise profiles of the nursing-home population are hard to sketch, but here are some facts gathered from a variety of studies. Nursing-home residents are overwhelmingly senior citizens. They are predominantly women (71 percent), widowed or widowers (62 percent), and white (92 percent). Only 12 percent are married. Most residents have significant physical and mental health problems: 48 percent suffer from arteriosclerosis; 35 percent have heart trouble; 32 percent suffer from mental disorientation; 25 percent suffer from chronic brain syndrome; 25 percent have arthritis and rheumatism; 21 percent have hypertension; 16 percent have suffered at least one stroke. Sadly, 50 percent have no immediate family or friends that visit them.

Nursing-home residents need help to get through each day. They need help bathing (85 percent); dressing (70 percent); using the toilet (more than 50 percent); and eating (more than 30 percent). The extent of dependency among nursing-home residents has been increasing. From 1979 to 1983, the portion of nursing-home residents with major dependencies has climbed from 77 percent to more than 90 percent. As elderly Americans become incontinent and dependent on personal assistance for basic functions like eating and using the toilet, it becomes extremely difficult to care for them at home.

There are two kinds of nursing homes. Skilled nursing facilities (SNFs) provide twenty-four-hour-a-day nursing services. They specialize in medically oriented nursing care, prescribed by a patient's physician and provided by registered nurses, licensed practical nurses, and nurses aides. They also provide restorative, physical, occupational, and other therapy. Both Medicare and Medicaid pay for skilled nursing care, although Medicare's coverage is limited to 100 days following hospitalization.

Intermediate care facilities (ICFs), which may coexist in the same home with skilled nursing facilities, provide less intensive medical, nursing, social, and rehabilitative services to people who are incapable of independent living, although they do not need continuing medical care. Medicaid covers intermediate care; Medicare does not. There are also intermediate care facilities for the mentally retarded.

Nationally, Medicare certifies 67 percent of skilled nursing facilities for use by its beneficiaries. Medicare certification is more important as a badge of quality than as a source of funds. Even among certified facilities, half have less than 5 percent of their patient-days paid by Medicare.

With occupancy pressing capacity, with thousands on nursing-home waiting lists, and with Medicaid's capped payment system, nursing homes prefer affluent "private pay" patients, those who can bear full charges with their own financial resources. Private pay patients, regardless of the level of care they require, usually have no difficulty in obtaining admission. Some homes require private pay patients to contract to remain so—i.e., not switch to Medicaid or Medicare—for periods ranging from six months to two years. Private pay patients are usually charged more, and homes do not have to maintain for them the detailed records Medicare and Medicaid require. This preference can aggravate the shortage of available beds. Because of high occupancy rates, nursing homes often find it economically more attractive to hold a few beds open until they can admit a person who can pay full dollar out of his or her own pocket. Nursing homes often maintain separate waiting lists for private, Medicare, and Medicaid patients.

After private pay patients, nursing homes prefer Medicaid beneficiaries who require relatively few services. Since most state Medicaid programs pay a flat, predetermined rate for nursing-home residents regardless of the care provided, homes naturally prefer individuals whose needs are few, particularly since Medicaid patients are more likely to stay longer. About 60 percent of Medicaid residents spend more than a year in the nursing home, whereas only 43 percent of private pay patients stay that long. Medicaid patients are twice as likely to spend five years or more in a nursing home as private pay patients.

Nursing homes that accept Medicare beneficiaries prefer those with the least difficult physical and social problems. Hospital administrators report that nursing-home operators seek to avoid heavy-care Medicare and Medicaid patients. The homes favor those who need well-defined therapies, like patients suffering from hip fractures and strokes; they shun those needing oxygen, skin care, and tube feedings. Even in the case of private payers, the homes have a tendency to avoid patients with severe emotional or mental problems.

Overall, the shortage of nursing homes is becoming more acute. One study found that more than 80 percent of staffed nursing facilities had waiting lists, with an average length of twenty-five names. By the year 2000, the number of Americans over seventy-five will have grown to more than 17 million. Those are the people who most need nursing-home care. As we had only about 1.5 million nursing-home beds in 1984, a massive construction program will be required, unless we find ways to increase the independence of the over-seventy-five population. On the basis of current utilization rates and lengths of stay, U.S. government agencies project that by the year 2000, there will be a need for at least 2.1 million nursing-home beds. That means that between 1985 and 2000—just fifteen years—an additional 600,000 beds would have to be constructed. One industry expert says that we need to build a 120-bed nursing home every day until the turn of the century. In 1984 each new bed represented a cost of $30,000; achieving the goal that year would have cost more than $1.3 billion.

We're not likely to get the new beds to meet the projected need. The same Medicaid program that created the industry has now gone full circle and is strangling its growth. To build a nursing home eligible for Medicaid reimbursement—an income-insurance policy most investors want—you must have permission from the state, in the form of a certificate of need. But Medicaid costs are driving state budgets into deficit, since states pay half the costs and the feds are increasingly reluctant to pay their share. So states see stopping or at least slowing the growth of nursing homes as a strategy for holding down their Medicaid spending, and they frequently delay or deny certificates of need to add more beds.

Often the shortage of nursing homes keeps patients in more expensive hospital beds. That's been fine for the states, as long as Medicare, fully funded by the feds, paid the bill. In 1983 the General Accounting Office reported that estimates of hospital "back-up days"—days spent in the hospital due to nursing-home bed shortages—ranged all over the lot: from 1 million to 9.2 million days, about 1 to 7 percent of all Medicare and Medicaid hospital days. At $400 to $500 dollars a day, the taxpayer is shelling out between $400 million and $4.6 billion to pay unnecessary hospital bills.

The DRG system is changing the pressures on hospitals, as we have seen. With Medicare DRGs providing an incentive to reduce the length of hospital stays (the predetermined payment for treating an illness is the same, however long the stay), hospitals are under increased pressure to discharge patients. This situation could intensify problems faced by Medicaid and Medicare patients in need of nursing-home care. Hospitals won't keep them, and nursing homes prefer to fill their beds with more profitable private pay patients and minimum-care Medicaid and Medicare patients. The frail elderly will be trapped in this vicious void.

How many nursing-home beds should we have?

The number of nursing-home beds per capita varies widely among the states, from a Florida low of 21.4 per 1,000 residents age sixty-five and over to a South Dakota high of 93.3. U.S. government analyses reveal that the more available beds are, the more they will be used.

There's no agreement on the appropriate number, because there's no consensus on what constitutes need, medical, social, economic or otherwise, for nursing-home care. Ultimately, the demand for such care rests on decisions made by individuals and families, often in consultation with physicians, other medical professionals, clergy, and social workers. These decisions involved not only the medical condition of an elderly person, and that person's ability to bathe, dress, feed, and toilet himself or herself, but also the capacities, financial and human, of the individual and his or her family to cope at home.

How these factors influence decisions varies. One family may use its income to provide services at home for an elderly family member, while another with equal income may purchase care for an elderly person as a private pay patient at a nursing home. For those with incomes sufficiently low to qualify for Medicaid, decisions about entering a nursing home can be affected by Medicaid's bias in favor of institutional care: its coverage of nursing-home costs is far more generous than its coverage of home health care. Only since the early 1980s has the Congress authorized Medicaid to experiment with reimbursement of community-based day care as a substitute for nursing-home care.

The impact of skewed financial incentives is apparent. We provide great incentives to put people in nursing homes with public dollars. We pump billions of research dollars into exotic machinery like artificial hearts and long-shot cancer therapies. But we skimp on reimbursement for home health care, we provide little incentive, through the tax code or otherwise, for families to take care of their own, we have ignored the potential of health promotion and disease prevention to keep our senior citizens independent as long as possible, and we have neglected to focus our scientific genius on extending the capacities of our senior citizens to take care of themselves independently.

The Golden Pond, where people can be self-sufficient and stay at home with some care, is the solution we should seek for most of our elderly, not the institutional nursing home. The reasons are not simply financial; indeed, the most important ones are human. Most people would much prefer to live in their homes and function independently than to endure the lethargy of institutionalized way stations on the road to death. Senior citizen centers in local communities are crowded with elderly people grateful for the opportunity to continue active social lives. We Americans should ease up on our obsession with extending breathing and heartbeats beyond eighty-five or ninety, whatever the cost, and turn our intellects, creativity, and energies to extending the independent capacities of our elderly.

The elderly bring into sharp focus the relationship between health care costs and a humane society. Nursing homes and Golden Ponds are just one part of it. The population explosion brought about widespread acceptance of birth control, and even abortion on demand, and in some parts of the world, involuntary sterilization. The combined force of a rapidly expanding elderly population and expensive medical technology may yet bring us death control if we do not get our priorities straight.

DEATH CONTROL

America is at the dawn of the first four-generation society in the history of the world. That dawn can be the start of a brilliant era in which great-grandfathers pass on a rich, living inheritance of love and wisdom to their great-grandchildren, or it can be the beginning of a frightening era of death control.

Which era dawns will depend on our moral values and compassion, and in large measure on our ability to create an efficient health care delivery system with its attention turned to keeping people well. Those who need and use our health care system most are the elderly, and those who pay most of the bill are the young workers of the "Me Generation." All the demographic portents are that fewer and fewer young people will have to pay for health care for more and more elderly ones.

As the twentieth century makes way for the twenty-first, we will become a society in which it will be common to have two generations of the same family in retirement, on Social Security, on Medicare, in the hospital. When a seventy-six-year-old patient of Jeanne Lynn, a Washington, D.C., geriatrician, died, she commented, "The real tragedy is that he'd been taking care of his ninety-five-year-old mother at home and now she has no one." Increasingly, those who take care of the elderly, particularly at home, will be elderly themselves.

The implications of this demographic transformation for our

nation are stunning in every aspect: voting patterns, shifts of political power, demands on economic resources and social service systems, housing, income redistribution. But nowhere is the aging of the American population more freighted with opportunity and danger than in the area of health care.

The issues of who lives and who dies, and at what cost, are complex and confounding. We must think deeply and with a long view if we are to comprehend them and deal with them wisely. But the omnivorous appetite of health care for our financial resources adds an urgency that demands action, under threat that our society will be torn apart by a debate over death control that will make the debate over abortion seem like genteel tea-party chatter. Unlike fetuses, the old can speak for themselves.

True, death control flies in the face of Judeo-Christian religion and ethics and the values of most civilized people. But just a little over a decade ago, so did abortion on demand. In that short time, our nation, despite its richness in Judeo-Christian tradition and teachings, has overturned law upon law and legalized about two million abortions a year, often financing them with public funds.

America is getting older. The decades since 1940 have seen a steady growth in the number of older citizens: a demographic change so large—and so striking—that it challenges all our systems for supporting the elderly, but especially and most insistently those that deliver health care.

Three dramatic and inexorable trends etch the aging of America:

First, life expectancy has increased by almost twelve years since 1940. In that year, the average life expectancy at birth was just over 63 years, lower than Social Security's retirement age of sixty-five. In 1985 life expectancy for all Americans is about seventy-five years: almost seventy-two for men, seventy-nine for women. In 1985 three-quarters of our population will reach age sixty-five. Once there, they will live, on the average, for another seventeen years, to age eighty-two. By the year 2050, we are told, life expectancy will increase only another four years for men and five for women. But healthier habits, better public health, biomedical advances, and increased access to health care have consistently rendered projections of life expectancy far too low.

Second, the postwar baby boom will result, early in the twenty-first century, in a senior boom. In 1940 roughly 7 percent of our people were sixty-five or over; today the proportion is about 12 percent, some 28 million. After 2010 the percentage of the elderly will soar, as the children of the baby boom grow old. By the year 2030, at least 21 percent of our population—66 million citizens—will be sixty-five or older.

Third, America's older population is itself aging. In 1940, less than 30 percent of people over sixty-five were seventy-five or older. By the year 2000, 50 percent of those over sixty-five will be seventy-five or older; more than 1 million Americans will be over ninety. Even in 1985, almost 12 million people, approximately 40 percent of Americans over sixty-five, are seventy-five or older.

The impact of this historically unprecedented aging of a nation acquires magnum force as a result of simultaneous trends in our society. Though people are living longer, they are retiring earlier; the birth rate is stabilizing at a lower level, and Americans are waiting to have babies at an older age. The erosion of the tax and support base is ominous. Thirty years ago, nearly one-half of all men sixty-five and over worked; in 1984, less than one man in five (and one woman in twelve) worked after age sixty-five. As baby-boomers swell the ranks of the elderly, the ratio of active workers to retired citizens will slip from about six to one in 1985 to about three to one in 2030.

The shift in the total dependent population—those under eighteen and over sixty-four—signals the menace ahead. In 1965, with the baby boom, there were almost four children under eighteen for each person over sixty-four. In 1985 the ratio is two children to each senior. By 2030 the ratio will be one to one, and shortly thereafter the number of elderly will exceed the youth population. For the health care system, this means fewer of the lowest-cost, lowest-intensity users of medical services, and lots more high-cost, high-intensity consumers—against the background of a shrinking proportion of active workers to pay the bills.

In 1984 Americans sixty-five and over used more than a third of the money we spent on personal health care, even though they comprised only 12 percent of the population. At almost twice that proportion of the population in the year 2030, if we go along as we have, those sixty-five and older will use two-thirds of the vastly increased dollars we'll spend for health care. Not only do basic medical costs rise, so does the need for home health assistance and nursing-home care. Only one out of twenty people between the ages of sixty-five and seventy-four needs help walking, while eight out of twenty people eighty-five years and older need such help.

The combination of the aging of our population, rising health care costs, and the shrinking proportion of actual workers is sobering and creates a financial and political crunch the likes of which our nation has never experienced. The money needed to keep Medicare's Hospital Insurance Trust Fund solvent is only the tip of the iceberg. Some thoughtful Americans see the Social Security crisis as a forerunner of far more frightening financial difficulties, as the nation encounters unfunded government and private-sector pension liabilities that may be close to $1 trillion.

But few Americans have even begun to think about the unfunded health care liability of our nation. In 1984 the unfunded postemployment health care cost liability of the Fortune 500 American companies alone—with about 15 million employees—approached $2 trillion. The total assets of those companies was only $1.4 trillion. That unfunded liability by itself reveals the severity of the financial and social crisis health care costs pose for this nation. And the revolution in health care technology provides the potential for sudden and geometric cost increases.

These monumental liabilities, the health care needs of a multiplying elderly population, and the potential cost of technology make it imperative to create an efficient health care delivery system. We can't keep going the way we are. We simply don't have the money. That stark fact presages a terrifying question of triage for the American people and an ugly debate over death control.

In *The Painful Prescription*, Henry Aaron and Dr. William Schwartz argue that, like Great Britain, America will soon ration health care. America has always had rationing, of course, related to individual economic wealth. But with Medicare and the Veterans Administration, government becomes the rationer for those who use and need acute care most. This role is reinforced by the fact that the federal government controls virtually all the basic biomedical research in America and, together with state and local governments, pays most hospital bills.

Bluntly put, Uncle Sam will soon be playing King Solomon with our fathers and mothers and with us.

Without the most energetic pursuit of efficiencies, America will soon be a nation in which there is no kidney dialysis for people over fifty-five and no hip operations (or artificial hips) for those over sixty-five; a nation in which eligibility for expensive anticancer therapy will be based on statistical assessments of success, and key organ transplants will be severely limited to special cases of virtually certain recovery—all as defined in pages and pages of government regulations and as understood in quiet compacts among bureaucrats and health care providers.

That seems a grim vision for the future of a country with the most miraculous medical complex in history. But in Great Britain that future is now. That is just about what the British have been doing.

Rationing started in Great Britain largely because its stagnant economy could not absorb major increases in health care costs. With virtually all hospitals owned by the government and virtually all doctors on government salaries, the British government is the only source of health care for most of its citizens. Although apparently on the rise, private spending pays for less than 5 percent of physician and hospital expenses and less than 12 percent of total health care. As the government weighs demands for health services against other public needs, such as defense, highways, education, and police protection, its decisions determine for most Britons what medical services they receive. Each of Britain's fourteen health regions (and each of their hospitals) gets a specific amount of money. If a region exceeds its budget in one period, the excess is subtracted from what it gets for the next. If prices go up more than expected, individual hospitals must make do within their budgets, if necessary postponing or even eliminating medical procedures and laying off doctors and nurses. Unless a case is urgent, a patient can wait weeks or months to see a specialist, months or even years to be admitted to a hospital. Of patients admitted to hospitals, one-third wait three months, 6 percent wait more than a year.

So the British National Health Service, which provides free health care, also rations what it provides, making choices about who will live and who will die. The British government treats less than half the cases of chronic kidney failure in England. Although kidney transplants take place at about the same rate as in the United States, kidney dialysis is performed at less than one-third the U.S. rate, and in substantially fewer cases than in other European countries. Since kidney failure is terminal, the decision not to provide dialysis is a sentence of death.

In Britain that decision, though not stated explicitly, is clearly related to the age of the patient. For its citizens up to age forty-four, Britain provides about the same level of treatment as France, West Germany, and Italy do, but for patients forty-five through fifty-four the rate of treatment slips to about two-thirds. British patients fifty-five through sixty-four receive treatment at only one-third the rate of treatment in the other three countries, and those over sixty-five are treated at less than one-tenth the rate. In the United States, virtually everyone with chronic kidney failure is treated, mostly under Medicare.

The British perform hip replacements at almost 80 percent of the U.S. rate, but patients wait an average of fourteen months, with some in line for years. Effectively, most over sixty-five are denied hip replacements. While there is a consensus that coronary bypass surgery is performed too often here in the United States, it is performed only one-tenth as often in Britain.

There's no point in saying it can't happen in America. It already is happening. In the early years of Medicare and Medicaid, government decisions invariably gave the old and the poor more medical services than had previously been available to them. In the early 1980s, spiraling health care costs collided with federal and state budgets hobbled by recession-driven deficits and, in the case of the federal budget, the people's desire for massive tax cuts. The old and the poor learned that the hand that caresses can also choke. The government started reducing medical services.

Predictably, rationing hit the poor first and hardest. Between 1981 and 1984, an estimated 700,000 children and 567,000 senior citizens lost Medicaid benefits. Some states sharply curtailed the number of hospital days, physician visits, and prescription drugs they would pay for.

Because Medicare serves the politically sophisticated elderly population, the government's steps in the direction of rationing services have been gingerly and indirect, through efforts to trim disability rolls and increase premiums, deductibles, and copayments. But attention is increasingly being given to not paying for high-cost, high-tech procedures. In 1980, after paying for heart transplants at Stanford University for six months, Medicare stopped reimbursements for the operations because of their expense and experimental status. In 1984 Medicare PROs started setting up prescreens for hospital admissions, a procedure that can deny surgery and other inpatient care to patients over their doctors' objections.

Medicare, the Veterans Administration, state health departments running Medicaid, and corporate employers and union leaders will soon face the same problems as those the British National Health Service has faced, unless we change our health care system. At no point is the issue likely to be presented in more wrenching or uglier manifestation than with the elderly.

The problem is as fundamental as ensuring that our towering technical brilliance has decent and not destructive effects, and as immediate as the last son or daughter who just told the doctor to disconnect a father or mother from the tubes through which the parent was breathing and eating. The urgency of informing our health care system with efficiency, or wringing from it billions of dollars of unnecessary hospitalization and waste, has far deeper roots than bankrupting Medicare, gobbling up larger shares of our gross national product, imposing higher taxes on our working population. The tap root of urgency goes to the morality and political civility of our society. Our failure as a people to confront and conquer the health care cost Goliath threatens all of us—and particularly the elderly—with a system of death control.

The seeds for such a system are already being planted. Dr. Paul Ellwood says that "we are nearing the day when we will have to confront the rationing of high-tech, very costly procedures." Dr. Schwartz believes that "the only way to cut costs will be to deny benefits to some people or deny benefits for some diseases." Colorado governor Richard Lamm says, "We're heading for a day when they can keep us alive long past when our quality of life is gone with transplants and high-technology medicine," and his reaction to this era of exotic and high-cost medicine is to tell the very ill elderly they "have a duty to die and get out of the way." As far back as the 1960s, a committee in Seattle, Washington, selected early patients for kidney dialysis based on their "value to society." Honeywell, Inc., approves, on an employee-by-employee basis, which will get reimbursed for heart, lung, or liver transplants. The Population Reference Bureau has expressed its concern that "the postponement of death increases federal costs, requiring more taxes."

In 1984 a grand jury in New York issued a blistering report about a hospital's "purple-dot system" to designate which terminally ill patients should be resuscitated and which should not. In response, Governor Mario Cuomo ordered the state health commissioner, Dr. David Axelrod, to write guidelines establishing under what circumstances doctors can deliberately let such patients die. Axelrod promised to recognize situations in which extraordinary methods "tend to prolong death rather than maintain life." In May 1985, Cuomo agreed to send to the state legislature a recommendation from Axelrod and the Governor's Task Force on Life and the Law that would require doctors to document the consent of a patient or surrogate (in the case of an incompetent patient) before intentionally letting a terminally ill patient die. Cuomo also agreed to draft health department rules setting out the procedures to be followed and defining death as "the irreversible cessation of all functions of the entire brain, including the brain stem."

Organ transplants that can make the difference between life and death have become a form of political patronage, with congressmen, governors, and even the President of the United States intervening to find organs and get Medicare and Medicaid to pay for operations. In actions that render the popular entertainment *Coma*—in which individuals were placed in a deep sleep and warehoused so their organs would be available for sale—something of a prophetic experience, Congress authorized the federal government to keep a computer file of available organs, and in 1985 New York State passed a law requiring hospitals to ask next of kin for organs of relatives at or near death. Patients and doctors are quarreling over the right to die and responsibilities to support life. The New Jersey Supreme Court first found that extraordinary means need not be deployed to sustain life, and later included nasogastric feeding, a common procedure, among the medical practices that could be discontinued for a terminally ill patient.

These questions are going to get harder, not easier. Who gets the next available liver? heart? lung? Who gets intensive care for how long? For every Governor Lamm, there's a Jacob Javits, speaking and lecturing while suffering from incurable Lou Gehrig's disease, and asking, "Why should a terminal illness be different from a terminal life?" Isn't the individual always entitled to stay alive as long as he or she can?

I am not suggesting that we can avoid these questions by tempering the advances of technology. Luddites in nineteenth-century England, who invaded textile factories and smashed machines because of their desperate opposition to technology, solved nothing in their day, and their descendants will solve nothing in ours. But we should insist that progress serve a decent human end, inform our scientific genius with morality, and recognize the moral dimension of our obligation to use our health care dollars effectively.

I do believe that we can have an America without a completely institutionalized, government-legislated, and bureaucrat-operated system of death control. We are fortunate because we still have time to avoid that fate. We can learn from Britain's experience. Our society is far more productive than Great Britain's. Our nation can well afford to provide quality medical care to all if we have the courage to act and the stamina and persistence to eliminate the profligacy of our health care system in the face of potent economic special interests.

If some sort of death control is to be an inevitable feature of American society, then we must prepare for it. We need time to plan, to think through the incredibly perplexing ethical, religious, and social issues, to work and agonize our way to a system of dignity, justice, and compassion, to assure the primacy of the person over machinery and technology. An efficient health care system can provide that critical time.

No matter how wise or efficient we are, we will still confront a host of ethical issues of the kind that lead moral theologians to thank God there's a God. Though our health care system remains—and, I believe, should remain—dominantly a private one, the cutting edge of many decisions is likely to be faced first through government programs. As government has financed health care and biomedical research, it has become the center of bitter controversies over what it should pay for, controversies that involve questions about when life begins, when it ends, and the nature of human existence.

Should government pay for all heroic life-extending measures? If not, when should it pay and when not? Does it make sense to allocate 30 percent of our multibillion-dollar Medicare bill to high-tech medical services for those who have less than a year to live?

The sagas of artificial heart recipients like Dr. Barney Clark and William Schroeder alert us to the probability that the geniuses of modern medicine and bioengineering will some day perfect for us a workable, artificial heart. But do we have the geniuses to decide who should be eligible to have such a marvelous, life-sustaining— and incredibly expensive—device?

Under what circumstances should extraordinary medical technology be withdrawn from—or granted to—terminally ill patients? Who makes that decision: a judge, a parent or spouse, a rich uncle, the executor of a living will or the holder of a durable power of attorney, a federal or state bureaucrat, a priest, a family doctor, a cancer researcher, a pediatrician, an emergency-room resident, the highly drugged, physically shattered, or emotionally distraught patient? Who among those is best equipped to draw the line between natural death, euthanasia, suicide, and murder?

Whoever makes the decision, can legislators, governors, Secretaries of Health and Human Services, medical administrators, corporate executives, union leaders, commercial insurers, and the Blues wash their hands like Pontius Pilate?

America cannot tolerate a health care system that wastes as much as $75 billion a year, when tighter corporate and government budgets force choices that may result in life for some and death for others.

No modern society, not even one as wealthy as our own, can completely escape the issues of death control. But we have the resources, if we apply them effectively, to keep government in its place, to make fewer hard choices necessary, and to concentrate our collective wisdom on those choices we truly cannot avoid. The tragedy will be if we continue to waste our health care dollars and resources by throwing them into a reimbursement system with little incentive for efficiency. The judgment of our parents, our children, history, and God could be harsh if we choose to squander our resources so profligately. That judgment could come in our lifetime, on our families, because the elderly are eventually ourselves and our children.

Chapter 11

SHAPING
THE REVOLUTION

So what can we do to arrest towering health care costs and pre-serve and enhance our miraculous medical system?

Plenty.

We can shape this incipient revolution into a fundamental transformation of the personal motivations, financial incentives, and institutional roles and relationships of doctors, hospitals, pa-tients, and purchasers of health care.

To do so, we've got to stop blaming the other guy—the patient, doctor, hospital administrator, health insurer, medical equipment manufacturer, drug company, malpractice lawyer, union, corpo-rate employer, government bureaucrat. All of us must look to our-selves, to what we can do differently. We must change the way we think about health care.

STAYING OUT OF THE SICK CARE SYSTEM

The first step is to recognize the difference between health care and sick care. We have been paying for a sick care system. Funda-mentally, we've provided too many financial incentives for doctors to treat us when we are sick rather than teach us how to stay well, to send us to the hospital rather than keep us out of it.

Physicians have become the repairmen of the system, hospitals and clinics are the shops they work in, and scanners, radiation, drugs, and scalpels are their tools. We use doctors when our bodies or minds break down. We've come to rely on their marvelous inventions to compensate for our excesses. We have forgotten the purpose of all those pills and medicines: to cure us when we are ill, not to give us the capacity to further abuse our bodies and minds. Tranquilizers, for example, are to help us when we have suffered too much stress, but far too often doctors give us Valium pills so we can subject ourselves to more stress.

Each of us can do more for our own health than any doctor, any hospital, any machine, or any drug.

Heart disease is America's number-one killer. Daily newspapers and television dramas give the impression that coronary bypass surgery, modern cardiopulmonary techniques, miracle hypertension pills, human heart transplants, and in the future, animal and artificial heart transplants are the way to battle heart disease.

Right?

Couldn't be more wrong.

Since 1970 our nation has experienced a dramatic 25 percent decline in deaths from coronary heart disease. The major reasons? Improved eating habits—the reduction in cholesterol—accounted for almost one-third of the drop. The decline in cigarette smoking was responsible for another quarter. So individuals, by changing personal habits, were responsible for more than half the decline in deaths from heart disease. In contrast, coronary care units accounted for only 13.5 percent; cardiopulmonary resuscitation, 4 percent; bypass surgery 3.5 percent; and the widely used hypertension pills only 9 percent. Deaths from stroke are also sharply down for much the same reasons.

Virtually all factors that substantially increase likelihood of heart disease are within the patient's, not the doctor's control: smoking, a high-cholesterol diet, other improper eating patterns, obesity, lack of exercise, stress. The other factors that increase risk are hypertension and diabetes, both of which are frequently caused and exacerbated by actions and life-styles within our control—and adult diabetes can be most effectively contained by proper diet if detected early.

America's number-two killer is cancer. What activity most increases the risk of getting this horrible disease? Cigarette smoking. Improper diet is also a big culprit.

Smoking is slow-motion suicide, a menace that has taken more American lives than all our wars and all our auto accidents combined, not only through heart disease and cancer, but through another two of the ten leading causes of premature death: influenza/pneumonia and accidents.

Alcohol is a grim reaper involved in five of the ten leading causes of untimely death in America: cancer, accidents (notably auto), cirrhosis of the liver, suicide, and homicide.

Even the fact that we leave dangerous stuff in the wrong places around the house—from toys on the stairs to poisons under the sink to open drug containers in the medicine cabinet—is among the leading causes of accidental injuries that require medical care and cause permanent disability and death.

So, not only for the chief causes of needlessly early death, but for many diseases and injuries as well, as Pogo teaches, we have met the enemy and they are us.

British Prime Minister Winston Churchill put it characteristically well on a visit to his personal physician because of headaches, wheezing, aches, pains, and shortness of breath. "You've got to stop smoking a dozen cigars a day and staying up half the night drinking a bottle of cognac," his doctor admonished. "If I wanted to do that," Churchill shot back, "I wouldn't need you."

These self-inflicted trips to the doctor and hospital are where the money goes. The total annual economic costs (including lost productivity) of heart disease and stroke are about $100 billion; of cancer, at least $50 billion; of accidents, poisoning, and violence, another $100 billion; of respiratory diseases, like bronchitis and emphysema, about $50 billion; and of digestive diseases, like cirrhosis of the liver, more than $50 billion. Smoking alone accounts for $24 billion just in health care costs; alcoholism and alcohol abuse, at least $15 billion—to say nothing of another $100 billion in disability payments and lost productivity.

Reducing health costs begins at home. Changing life-styles—particularly with respect to smoking, excessive drinking, improper diet, and lack of exercise—offers the greatest opportunity for cutting costs. In a free country, pursuit of a healthy life-style is voluntary. But we can certainly take a host of actions to encourage Americans to choose wisely, and to bear the cost when they don't.

Health education should be required in every school in the country, beginning in the earliest grades. State and local education boards should make such courses as compulsory as reading and mathematics. The subjects covered should include everything from basic health habits, like brushing teeth, reducing sugar intake, and using over-the-counter medicines properly, to intensive teaching about the dangers of cigarette smoking, alcohol and drug abuse, and teenage pregnancy and sexually transmitted diseases. Health education should begin in preschool and continue in each of the twelve years of elementary and high school, and be integrated with compulsory physical exercise programs. It should become more sophisticated as each year progresses, building on prior learning, like reading, spelling, and math. Schools should teach how to use self-health products, such as kits that allow individuals to determine their sugar levels, take their own blood pressure, and perform other tests, thus becoming aware of their own health and being able to report to their doctors over the phone. Physical education instructors should teach health behavior and use calisthenics to give pupils an understanding of how the cardiopulmonary system works.

Each public elementary and secondary school should have a nurse, full-time if the enrollment is sufficiently large, part-time (perhaps shared with another school) if the enrollment is smaller. This paramedical can teach, spot the first signals of drug and alcohol abuse, provide early treatment, assist social workers and teachers with problem children, get visual and hearing problems identified early, alert teachers to high-risk students, such as children of alcoholics. Particularly in poor urban and rural areas, where most (sometimes all) children are on welfare and most mothers of children in the early grades are in their late teens and twenties, a school nurse can be as important as any teacher.

Colleges should make health education a part of their core curriculum, requiring at least one or two courses over the four-year period and physical education for all students not engaged in athletics. Particularly in the last two years of high school and in college, such education should teach how to: select doctors, get second opinions on elective surgery and nonmaternity, nonemergency hospital admissions, check bills and charges—in short, how to be informed and skeptical buyers in the sick care part of the health care system.

Health promotion and education should continue throughout the working careers of our citizens. Each company of any significant size should provide ample opportunities, as many now do, for workers to get proper exercise. They should also use their employee publications to keep workers informed on the importance of healthy habits. They should adopt health care insurance plans that encourage employees to pursue healthy life-styles and reward those who do. For example, employees who do not smoke should pay less for health and life insurance coverage than those who do. Several companies offer such policies, with big savings for health and disability insurance for nonsmokers.

As is the case with individuals, a major role of federal, state, and local government in holding down health care costs is to promote healthy life-styles. Government's responsibility extends not only to influencing individual behavior and reviewing the efficacy and safety of drugs and medical devices, but also to regulation of segments of modern society that increase the risks of America's top killers and cripplers. Some of government's most important work lies outside the sick care system of doctors, hospitals, machines, and medicines. Government has a pivotal role to play in accident prevention: by eliminating the easy availability of handguns, enacting tough drunk-driving laws; influencing the design of automobiles and motorcycles; requiring compulsory seat belt laws, highway speed limits, and safe roadway design and lighting. In cancer prevention, government plays a critical role in enforcing clean air and clean water laws, controlling environmental contaminants and chemical wastes, and setting and enforcing tough safety standards for the workplace. These tasks can be carried out without burdensome regulations.

Smoking offers a good example of the kind of society-wide effort required if we are serious about building a health care system that avoids unnecessary sick care costs.

Government and public health authorities have been alerting people to the dangers of smoking for years, and there are substantial indications that millions have been listening. But the accumulating evidence about the dangers of involuntary, second-hand smoking requires a new set of government responses. Studies in Japan, Germany, Hong Kong, Greece, Scotland, and the United States point to a clear relationship between exposure to other people's cigarette smoke and lung cancer. An Environmental Protection Agency researcher has found that tobacco smoke breathed by nonsmokers kills up to 5,000 of them each year and poses a larger cancer risk than all industrial air pollutants. An American Cancer Society study found that nonsmoking women who live with men who smoke a pack of cigarettes a day are twice as likely to get lung cancer as those who live with nonsmokers.

In October 1984, U.S. Surgeon General Dr. C. Everett Koop wrote that "there is all the medical evidence necessary" to protect the nonsmoker against "the irritation and potential harm that comes from other people's smoke." Koop noted that "pollution from tobacco smoke in homes, offices, other worksites, and in certain public places can reach levels which exceed contaminant levels permitted under environmental and occupational health regulations." Because Koop is concerned about the increasing evidence "that environmental tobacco smoke can bring about disease, including lung cancer, in healthy persons, including infants and children," he advises nonsmokers "to avoid exposure to cigarette smoke wherever possible" and particularly urges that children and infants be protected from involuntary smoking.

We should declare our elementary and secondary schools smoke-free zones, thus making them beacons for the first generation of a smoke-free society. Smoking should be prohibited in all enclosed public places, not simply because of the danger to others from secondary smoking, but because the more difficult it is for smokers to puff away, the more often they are reminded of the danger of their addiction, the likelier they are to quit. Local public authorities can also recognize the right of each person to smoke-free space at work, in public buildings like convention halls and auditoriums, and in other places open to the public, like restaurants and hotels, which can set aside smoke-free areas, rooms, and floors for diners and lodgers.

Any nonsmoker who has had the pleasure of eating in a smoke-free section of a restaurant knows how wonderful it is. Restaurants that provide such space, voluntarily or under local ordinance, report enthusiastic customer acceptance. Anyone who has opened the door to a smoke-stenched hotel room appreciates those hotels that set aside no-smoking accommodations.

The number of states that have overcome the well-bankrolled efforts of the tobacco lobby and restricted smoking in public places has been steadily rising. By 1985, twenty-eight states limited or banned smoking in health facilities, seventeen states restricted smoking in public buildings, fourteen in restaurants, eleven in government workplaces, and eight in private workplaces. Scores of towns, cities, and counties have enacted such laws, even in states that have not yet moved to restrict smoking in enclosed spaces. The self-serving advertising campaign of the Reynolds Tobacco Company against smoke-free space attests to the impact of such policies in reducing smoking. The issue is not smokers' rights. The issues are whether we intend to protect nonsmokers from involuntarily breathing tobacco smoke, whether we care enough about our fellow human beings who smoke to encourage them to stop killing themselves, and whether we're serious about the billions of dollars of health care costs smoking causes.

All modes of local public transportation should prohibit smoking. Airlines should certainly prohibit it, for pilots and crews and for all passengers during all flights. No smoking should be allowed on the ground when there are take-off delays.

Employers should establish no-smoking policies in the workplace. As Secretary of HEW, I issued an order requiring that each employee's right to smoke-free space be recognized. After a few shakedown weeks, all employees, smokers and nonsmokers alike, not only lived with it, they reported that they were much happier than before. In April 1984, Malcolm T. Stamper, president of the Boeing Company, established a corporate policy to create a smoke-free workplace. As an initial step, Boeing prohibited smoking in common areas throughout the workplace, such as hallways, restrooms, lobbies, libraries, and computer rooms. When Stamper first put this policy in place, he expected resistance from the workers and the union. Instead he got acceptance and appreciation. Many companies are strictly limiting smoking to designated areas. Workplace no-smoking policies make health and business sense,

because smokers are significantly less productive and far more ac-
cident- and illness-prone than nonsmokers. So anything that encourages people not to smoke at all and prohibits them from
puffing on the job will cut health care costs.

The National Advisory Council on Drug Abuse in 1985 called
for laws to ban all advertising of cigarettes, and all promotion
through tournament sponsorship or free distribution to young
Americans at concerts to get them hooked. Noting the deaths and
disease from smoking, the council condemned "the flood of cigarette advertising . . . in our print media." The tobacco industry's
$2.5 billion 1983 budget, a 36 percent increase over 1982, demon-
strates the importance it attaches to advertising to get Americans
more addicted to tobacco. Athletes should refuse to participate in
tournaments sponsored by cigarette companies. By what calcula-
tion of greed and cynicism do female tennis pros play in a tournament sponsored by Virginia Slims, the Philip Morris, Inc., brand
that seeks to lure young women into smoking, when thanks to
smoking, lung cancer in 1985 surpassed breast cancer as the number-one cancer-killer?

Newspaper and magazine publishers have an important responsibility here. Cigarettes are the only legally salable product in
America whose intended use kills and maims. Yet only a few major
publications, such as *Reader's Digest, The New Yorker, Christian
Science Monitor, Good Housekeeping, Saturday Evening Post*, and
Seventeen, refuse to accept cigarette advertising. Other major
publications rail against the dangers of smoking and attack the hy-
pocrisy of a government policy that urges us not to smoke yet sub-
sidizes farmers to grow tobacco. But these same newspapers and
magazines are just as hypocritical: they not only run cigarette ads,
they hustle to get them, and they refuse to carry ads alerting people to the dangers of smoking.

The *New York Times* has run its own advertising in the *U.S. Tobacco and Candy Journal* soliciting cigarette ads: "Life-styles are
made, not born" reads one of their cynical salutations. This *Times*
ad, published in January 1984, goes on to put the prestige of the
Times news and editorial columns at the disposal of the cigarette
companies: "Three million weekday readers and four million Sun-
day readers *believe* in the trend-setting advertising they see in its

atmosphere of quality and credibility" (emphasis in original ad). *Cosmopolitan* refused to carry an ad for antismoking clinics for fear of offending its cigarette advertisers.

In 1983 *Newsweek*, which, according to the Council on Science and Health, carried an average of ten full-page cigarette ads per issue, bringing in $750,000 each week, wouldn't permit an American Medical Association health care supplement to attack smoking, for fear of offending its cigarette advertisers. A year later, in October 1984, *Time* published a supplement, "Strategies for a Healthier, Happier and Longer Life," developed by the American Academy of Family Physicians. According to the Academy, *Time* edited the text, which originally contained many strong statements on the dangers of smoking, to such an extent that it "blunted, short-circuited and impaired the credibility of [the supplement] by cutting out all narrative references to smoking." The only caution on smoking that survived *Time*'s dollar-hungry censors was the admonition not to smoke in bed.

Ms. magazine pushes cigarettes to its women readers with glamorous full-color ads issue after issue, callously ignoring in its grab for advertising dollars the cancer and heart disease smoking causes among women—and the grim fact that women who smoke like men die like men who smoke.

Newspapers and magazines that hawk cigarettes should not be able to camouflage their avarice by talking fatuous First Amendment rights. The right claimed here is the freedom to push tobacco, one of our nation's most addictive and deadly drugs, which kills 360,000 Americans a year. If the First Amendment didn't stop *Newsweek* and *Time* from keeping antismoking material out of health supplements, then it shouldn't be invoked as a reason for them to refuse to run tobacco company ads. Newspapers that editorialized against the Vietnam War for its senseless killing might want to contemplate the far greater number of Americans who die each year from smoking the cigarettes they advertise.

Dealing with cigarette addiction won't be easy. William Pollin, director of the National Institute of Drug Abuse, calls tobacco "a powerfully addictive drug, deadlier than any other, eight times more addictive and four times deadlier than excessive use of alcohol, and much harder to treat than heroin addiction." But the payoff here is big: a 10 percent decrease in per capita cigarette consumption would avert more than 11,000 premature deaths a year; the savings in health care costs from such a drop would exceed $1 billion. And so is the opportunity: the drop in total cigarette consumption in 1982 and 1983—by 8 percent in the latter year alone—indicates that alerting people to the dangers of smoking works. The sharpest drops have been among men and those with a college education. Future campaigns should target young women (in the age group from eighteen to twenty-four their rate of smoking exceeds men's) and the less educated.

Alcohol represents a more subtle but no less important challenge. With cigarettes, the object is to get people to stop using them entirely. With alcohol, the goal is moderation. Nevertheless, many of the same principles apply. Particularly for teenagers, out of sight, out of mind is a good start. There should be no advertising of beer or wine on television and no advertising of liquor, beer, or wine with glamorous individuals, like athletes or entertainers. Since 1954 the U.S. Bureau of Alcohol, Tobacco, and Firearms has prohibited professional athletes from appearing in wine, beer, and liquor ads. This prohibition should apply not only during their professional careers but for ten years thereafter. Eventually, to the extent permitted, all alcohol and cigarette advertising, as well as ads for smokeless tobacco, should be limited to tombstone ads, without any human beings, a policy Britain applies to cigarettes. Laws raising the drinking age to twenty-one, strictly enforced, and rigorous punishment, including mandatory jail sentences, of drunk drivers can have a major impact on death and disability and the accompanying health care costs.

Immunization can keep millions of individuals out of the sick care system. Public health authorities bear the heaviest responsibility here, particularly with respect to children and high-risk adults. For children, no program has a higher payoff in cost-effectiveness than immunization. The cost-to-savings ratio is big not only for polio vaccination, but for vaccination against measles, whooping cough (pertussis), diphtheria, tetanus, and mumps as well. Every dollar spent on childhood immunization saves ten dollars in medical costs. When I became Secretary of Health, Education, and Welfare in 1977, only 65 percent of our school-age children were immunized against these diseases. We mounted a major program to get more than 90 percent immunized by 1979. Since then, the portion of children immunized has not increased significantly—and in 1984 the number of measles cases jumped 69 percent over the 1983 total—largely because the federal government has not purchased and distributed enough vaccine and because of failure of many state and local leaders to enforce strictly laws requiring immunization of all school-age children. With a vigorous childhood immunization program, we can wipe out measles as an indigenous disease in the United States in three years. Can anyone doubt the value of such investment in terms of health care costs—and averted human suffering?

Similarly, public health authorities should establish a system for flu and pneumonia immunization, through vaccines, for all adults over sixty-five and those under sixty-five with chronic respiratory diseases. For a modest investment, we can save millions of dollars in medical costs and avoid utterly unnecessary human suffering, incapacitation, and death. Part of any federal immunization program for children or high-risk adults should respond to the legitimate concerns of vaccine manufacturers about liability for adverse reactions, a tiny number of which are inevitable, and costly, despite the exercise of due care.

THE PATIENTS

To a great degree, the American health care system is consumer driven. Doctors and hospitals give patients what they want under the circumstances they find themselves in. Patients want everything that might conceivably provide cure or relief of symptoms, whatever the cost, especially when they're not paying. So the consumer, as well as the doctor and hospital, must become cost-conscious; this will ease some of the pressures patients place on doctors to provide unnecessary services and will encourage patients to seek efficient care. Where consumers have been paying for health care themselves, prices have risen less rapidly and patients have been less likely to seek unneeded care. This has been the case, for example, with over-the-counter pharmaceuticals.

There are a variety of ways to bring home the cost of unnecessarily expensive health care: taxing employee health benefits above a certain amount, requiring deductibles and copayments in public and private reimbursement plans, offering financial rewards (such as the elimination of deductibles or copayments) for those who select efficient plans. It's not necessary to select one over another. Combinations may make sense. At this stage in the revolution, a variety of methods should be tried. The critical objective is to make the consumer aware that different health care choices carry different costs. Then the consumer—government, business, individual patients—will reclaim the right, surrendered long ago, to deal only with efficient health care sellers. As we exercise this right, we will see vast changes in the attitudes and efficiency of hospitals and doctors. Gone will be the seller's market, where the real buyer never sees the bill.

In making Americans conscious of the cost of health care, we must be careful not to deter individuals, particularly the needy, from seeking necessary treatment. As HEW Secretary, I helped finance a series of studies of the impact of cost sharing, to be conducted over several years by the Rand Corporation. The jury is still out, but we are learning a great deal from these Rand studies. For example, there is some evidence that making health care free can help the poor, but does encourage excessive use of the system by others. A five-year study of 2,000 families revealed that on the whole, free medical services for children raised medical costs by one-third without any across-the-board health improvements, although such services seemed to improve the health of poor children with anemia and hearing difficulties. A study of a group of adults found that free medical care reduced the severity of hypertension especially among the poor. The early experience of corporations which have increased copayments and deductibles is that use of the health care system drops without any impact on the health of employees. At least initially, it appears that some degree of cost sharing for those able to pay may help reduce unnecessary use of health care professionals and facilities without adversely affecting their health. The concept may be most effectively deployed by requiring cost sharing for patients who choose less efficient delivery systems, but not for those who choose more efficient ones—just as most plans require patients who choose private rooms to pay the extra cost. But cost sharing for the poor seems unwarranted.

The American patient must become an informed consumer. Central to a free market with few controls and a variety of payment systems for physicians, hospitals, and other suppliers is an informed purchaser of medical services.

It is imperative to get lots of information out: what doctors charge, how successful they are in handling different types of patients, what kinds of diseases they treat most frequently, how often they use drugs or resort to hospitalization or surgery for particular diseases.

Doctors oppose the release of information like this. (They successfully blocked publication of the amount of taxpayer money each doctor collected in Medicare fees when I was Secretary of HEW.) They argue that to release such information is unfair, because doctors who treat difficult patients will have lower success rates (but any statistics released can indicate the severity of the cases treated), violates patient privacy (but there's no need to reveal patient names), will mislead the public, because only doctors are well enough educated medically to understand such information (but that depends how the information is disseminated). These are arguments always propounded to protect secrecy—whether civilian bureaucrats, corporate executives, military officers, or diplomats are making the case. It's much easier for the doctors, governors, board chairmen, generals, and ambassadors to do their work in secret. But it's not the doctors' lives we're supposed to make easy. It's ours we are trying to make and keep healthy—at a reasonable cost.

Patients should also get more information about hospital charges. In Minneapolis–St. Paul, at least thirty hospitals publish average prices for treating various medical ailments. Price alone is not enough. Under a 1985 Department of Health and Human Services regulation, peer review organizations under contract with Medicare will publish information about outcomes, lengths of stay, methods of treatment, and hospital-acquired infections, by category of disease. In view of the shocking revelations of variances in treatment covered in this book and so many other studies, the importance of such information is clear. Armed with it, patients and corporate purchasers will be able to make the kinds of informed choices about their hospitals that they have traditionally made about far less significant purchases. Comparable information should be made available on doctors' performances.

THE MEDICINE MEN

Doctors have by and large neglected their responsibility in health promotion and disease prevention. To get costs under control, doctors must focus on keeping us healthy. That's the work we should, in the first instance, train and pay them to do.

We can't change the health care system without the cooperation of its high priests, the doctors, any more than official Catholic doctrine can be changed without the approval of the Pope and his cardinals. Medical schools and professors influence the attitudes of doctors. They should imbue their students with their responsibilities to keep patients healthy, to seek the least expensive treatment, to recognize symptoms of addiction, and to use effective resources outside the old-boy doctor-hospital health care system. Programs like Harvard's New Pathway curriculum should be tried by other medical schools.

Far more time and training should be devoted to teaching medical students how to recognize and then treat America's most pervasive cause of illness and accident: addiction—whether to alcohol, cigarettes, other drugs, like marijuana, cocaine and heroin, or pills like Valium, barbiturates, and sedatives.

Medical schools should train students, and prod practitioners, to count to ten before employing spectacular—and extraordinarily expensive—technology, whatever the marginal benefit, beyond the point at which it fosters the mental, spiritual, and physical capacity or human dignity of the patient, and teach them to be more skeptical in resorting to surgery and less promiscuous in dispensing pills.

Medical academia should lead the way in changing doctors' attitudes about geriatric care. Much more attention should be placed on raising the quality of life and increasing the self-sufficiency of the elderly. To achieve this requires a sea change in the outlook of the medical profession (and indeed society itself), which medical schools are uniquely positioned to lead.

Americans seventy-five and over are the nation's fastest-growing age group. For them, our focus should be self-sufficiency into later years, giving the elderly more satisfying lives and rendering them less likely to need expensive health care and custodial services. Physicians should be trained to press health promotion and disease prevention for this population, to keep Americans seventy-five and over out of hospitals and nursing homes, rather than to commit them to such expensive care and then run their medical money-meters on bedside visits. A 15 percent reduction in the number of Americans between seventy-five and eighty-five requiring custodial care or hospitalization by 1990 could save up to $10 billion annually.

State and private accreditation authorities can require that medical schools change their curricula to cover these subjects adequately. On licensing exams, they can include questions on addiction prevention and treatment, geriatric care, health promotion, and cost-effective treatment, to help ensure that new doctors have greater knowledge and sensitivity in these areas.

It's also critical to change the financial incentives of doctors. When we buy a car, the manufacturer gives us a warranty that it will work for a certain period; if it doesn't, the manufacturer fixes it without charge. To stay eligible for the warranty, we must take care of our car, service it, get the oil changed, use unleaded gasoline, get periodic checkups.

There's an analogy here for reshaping America's health care system so that we pay doctors and dentists to tell us how to keep healthy. We would have to follow their guidance, of course, and if we didn't, we would have to pay the price, just as we would if our car engine broke down because we failed to lubricate it.

How would such a system work?

For doctors. We would pay our family physicians a certain amount each year to give us the proper tests and physical exams, to tell us a proper weight range and, if necessary, set up a diet to get us within that range and help us stay there, to prescribe minimum exercise programs for each member of the family, to watch our cholesterol levels, to provide family-planning (sex education) advice, and to treat routine illnesses and injuries, like colds, flus, stomach upsets, sprains, pulled muscles, and minor broken bones.

For our part, we would have to follow the doctors' advice—or pay more to the insurance company or Blue Cross/Blue Shield. If a family member smoked, the annual payment would be higher. The payment would also be increased for obesity, for not bringing down high cholesterol levels within a reasonable time, for excessive drinking of alcoholic beverages, and for failure to get the appropriate physical exams and tests.

For dentists. We would pay the dentist a set fee each year for all dental care. There would be additional charges only if patients did not fulfill their part of the contract. If children in the high-cavity years—say ages five to seventeen—did not report for periodic fluoridation treatment, there would be a charge for each missed treatment. If an adult missed a periodic checkup, there would be a charge. If a certain number of checkups were missed consecutively, the individual would be dropped from this plan and forced into a more expensive payment system.

Such arrangements with doctors and dentists can truly be called health care contracts; they are in sharp contrast to the sick care fee-for-service arrangements, under which all the economic incentives for physicians are to provide services for patients after they are sick (or think they're sick).

What happens under this system when a patient follows the rules but nevertheless gets seriously ill and requires surgery, hospitalization, treatment for heart disease or cancer? Such care would be provided, and paid for, under an insurance arrangement that assessed no fault to the doctor or the patient. But the family physician would be called upon to perform one more function: the role of gatekeeper and case manager. It would be his responsibility to lead the patient through the labyrinth of health care specialists. Only if the family doctor made (or should have made) the referral to a specialist would the patient be reimbursed for the cost of such care.

The importance of getting the family physician to concentrate on his responsibilities of health promotion, disease prevention, and case management with his patients is underscored by a preliminary analysis of Chrysler's 1984 health care data. In 1984, 3.4 percent of Chrysler's insured employees, retirees, and dependents accounted for 43.5 percent of the company's health care payments! (Sixty-three thousand of the 163,000 insured in Michigan made no claims for health care benefits.)

Our review of the cases of this high-cost 3.4 percent reveals that they are predominantly life-style-related diseases and that millions of dollars were wasted—and ineffective care provided—because no one was managing the care of these patients and aggressively pressing them to change their life-styles. More than half of the high-cost patients suffered from cancer, heart disease, respiratory illness, stomach and liver ailments, mental health problems, and alcohol or drug dependence identified as such. As we've seen, these problems are frequently attributable to cigarette smoking, alcohol or other substance abuse, improper diet, and inability to handle stress—all life-style factors that a health-care- rather than a sick-care-oriented family physician would focus on.

Once the Chrysler-insured patients were in the health care system, there was little medical management. For example, an alcohol-dependent patient got no follow-up after drying out and a month of rehabilitation therapy, so he returned for another round of the same treatment in less than six months. Patients were allowed to linger for weeks and die in hospitals when care could have been more appropriately, inexpensively, and humanely provided in a hospice or at home. Lack of patient care management also resulted in widespread unnecessary use of specialists.

Under a system where the doctor's role is to keep us healthy and self-referrals to specialists are not eligible for third-party reimbursement, the occasions for such treatment would be far less frequent and the amount of money spent on unnecessary specialized care would plummet.

Doctors who do not want to practice on a prepaid plan should be paid under a fee-for-illness system, not a fee-for-service one. The extravagant arrangement of paying a fee for each service a doctor performs encourages services even when they are of marginal benefit, or none at all. Under a fee-for-illness system, doctors would be paid a fixed amount to treat a patient for a particular illness—chicken pox, a winter flu, gastrointestinal infection, a broken arm—rather than a fee for each service performed, for example, each office visit, each home call, each examination. There would be variations, where relevant to the cost of treatment, similar to those in the DRG hospital system, for differences in age, complications, and geographic area; and there would be an appropriate payment scheme for chronic diseases like diabetes or hypertension. But the basic measure of payment would be the illness, not the service. The fee-for-illness system would cover the family physician, as well as surgeons' and specialists' charges not included in the DRG hospital payment.

As a first step, DRGs should be established to cover physicians' fees for inpatient hospital care. As with Medicare's hospital DRGs, a physician DRG system would set in advance a flat payment for all medical and surgical services provided during a hospital stay. This single payment could be made to the hospital or admitting physician, and either could then divide it among the doctors involved. It would cover the fees of the admitting doctor, surgeon, assistant surgeon, anesthesiologist, consulting specialists—regardless of how many doctors were involved or what services were performed. Doctors would thus have the same incentives as do hospitals under Medicare DRGs to perform only such services as are necessary for the good health of the patient. As with hospital DRGs, there would be variations related to particular cases.

At the same time, government, the Blues, and commercial insurers should work out the details of extending the fee-for-illness system to ambulatory care. In addition to establishing appropriate diagnosis groups and payment levels, such a system should have safeguards to stem unjustified creep to higher-intensity diagnoses that would entitle the doctor to greater fees. A fee-for-illness system will require less bureaucracy and paperwork, and less regulation, than one which pays fees for each service and must monitor thousands of schedule codes for those services, and it would give physicians an incentive to treat illnesses and injuries efficiently.

It will take time to develop such a system. In the interim, Medicare and other third-party payers should sharply reduce the thousands of schedule codes used to pay physicians for particular services, and not simply replace the "reasonable," "customary," and "prevailing" fee reimbursement system with uniform fees for each service. In the short run, caps on fees may offer some relief, but my experience as Secretary of HEW and as chairman of Chrysler's health care committee has been that when the government or the Blues set a payment cap on the fee for a particular service, the doctors create more services, and many simply perform the same service more often. Perhaps this is inevitable in a noncompetitive environment. The eventual reaction of the government or insurer is to establish new schedule codes for each service the doctors create, to require physicians to make the case for any service that is not on a code for treating a particular illness before paying for it, and to establish limits on how frequently a physician will be reimbursed for performing the same service. As a result, Medicare, the Blues, and private insurers have schedule codes for more than 6,000 specific procedures related to particular diagnoses, up from 2,000 in 1966, and they devise all sorts of computer programs and bureaucracies to detect physicians who perform the same services too often. Simply combining (in many cases recombining) similar or related codes would greatly reduce the profitable proliferation of medical procedures that generate unnecessary costs and risks to patients.

THE TEMPLES OF THE MEDICINE MEN

The objective should be to eliminate half the hospital beds in America. We can reduce the number of hospital beds by at least 30 percent by 1990, and another 20 percent by 1995. The Medicare DRG payment system is off to a good start. There is evidence that some patients are being moved out of hospitals too soon—and the PROs should carefully watch this—but overall, at significant reductions in costs, we are seeing care of the same or higher quality delivered with less risk. Hospital lengths of stay for Medicare patients and others are down. As the DRG system prompts more efficiencies, the staff-to-patient ratio should also begin to come down, approaching two to one from almost four to one.

Medicare's DRG system or others, such as preferred providers, flat-fee, direct-contract arrangements between companies and hospitals, health maintenance organizations, and salaried doctors, should be adopted by state Medicaid programs, the Blues, and commercial and self-insurers. Otherwise, hospitals will find ways to shift excessive and unnecessary costs to non-Medicare patients and the incentive for efficient treatment will be diluted.

The DRG system provides incentives to treat patients efficiently once they are in the hospital. To assure a 50 percent reduction in beds, we also need ways to keep out people who shouldn't be there. No one should be admitted to a hospital, except for maternity or emergency cases, without getting a second opinion from a disinterested doctor. This kind of hospital screen is proving effective in the experience of an increasing number of corporations and in Medicare demonstrations. Chrysler and Owens-Illinois have found reductions of 15 percent and more in hospital admissions of their insured employees and retirees where they have put such a program in place. Other means, such as denying payment for hospitalization unless approved by a professional review organization or insurance carrier, may be even more efficient. In the first six months of such a Medicare program in Kentucky, the number of hospital admissions dropped by 20 percent. As the Medicare peer review organizations analyze variations in treatment patterns, even sharper reductions will occur.

Our people and health care professionals must come to regard hospitals as what they really are: expensive institutions of last resort. Many surgical procedures performed in hospitals can be just as effectively and far less expensively performed in doctors' offices, neighborhood clinics, and outpatient surgical centers. Massachusetts General, one of our nation's premier hospitals, performs 200 kinds of operations on an outpatient basis at a cost 75 percent less than the cost of surgery involving a two-day admission. If we provide the same (or better) insurance coverage for a procedure performed outside the hospital, say, in the doctor's office, many surgical procedures and virtually all preadmission hospital testing can be done in nonhospital settings.

This will accelerate the arrival of the doctor's office of the future, which should be far more versatile and directly competitive with hospitals than is the office of today. With modern technology, physicians can perform in their offices many surgical and other procedures now done in hospitals, and effectively compete with hospitals and with freestanding surgical centers. With such offices, the continued growth of outpatient surgery centers, and our focus on health care rather than sick care, we can reduce the number of hospital beds in America from 4.2 to 2.1 or less for each 1,000 people. Many excess hospital beds can be diverted to ease long-term care problems that hover over the graying American population. Those that can't should be shut down to avoid shifting greater costs to fewer patients.

RESEARCH

America spends vast sums to install artificial hearts, transplant vital organs, and battle a legion of diseases. The miracles of modern medicine and the relief of human pain and suffering make many of those investments worthwhile.

But we don't spend nearly enough research money to learn more about the least expensive ways to achieve a particular medical outcome. As we've seen, there are wide variations in the type and cost of treatment for common ailments, like gall bladder problems, hypertension, tonsillitis, and heart disease. In one city there will be far more operations than in another—sometimes ten or even twenty times the surgery rate in one part of a state as compared with another—in treating identical symptoms in similar patients. Yet the return to health appears the same, and surgery may be thousands of dollars more expensive and far riskier to the individual, who sometimes suffers complications or contracts another ailment as a result of hospitalization. Too often the dominant determinant of the rate of surgery in a community has been the number of surgeons there: the more surgeons, the more surgery. We should determine what procedures, in similar circumstances, truly affect the medical outcome. Some such work is going on, but far more needs to be done. A commitment of millions to research here is likely to yield billions in savings and better-quality care.

Our publicly funded research efforts and the research of the medical equipment corporations should be more attentive to reducing the cost of medical care. The point is not to retard technology but to encourage it and ensure that advances are used efficiently. In a system of third-party, cost-based reimbursement, hospitals have not had sufficient incentive to relate costs of new inventions to benefits. Medical researchers and innovators, particularly in the exotic procedures and diagnostic equipment areas, have had little incentive to consider the cost-effectiveness of their dazzling magic. Medicare DRG hospital rates should not have a special additional component to pay for new technology. Like other businesses, the health industry should be required to finance such spending on the basis of the benefits to be achieved for the costs incurred.

The potential of turning our technological genius to cost-saving medical devices is enormous. The kidney-stone crusher can eliminate the need for 80,000 surgical operations at a fraction of the cost—if we can limit the number of crushers sold to the one hundred units we need as a nation. New laser techniques can revolutionize heart and eye surgery and cancer diagnosis and curtail the need for expensive hospitalization. A computer support system permits emergency-room attendants to use a hand-held calculator to determine in twenty seconds whether someone is suffering a heart attack; in early tests it has reduced by 30 percent the number of emergency-room cases admitted to expensive inpatient hospital care. A 1985 breakthrough in genetic engineering may produce a vaccine to eliminate malaria from the earth.

In the absence of a competitive system that keeps the attention of our medical technology companies on cost-effectiveness, we need an office of technology assessment to make determinations, certainly for Medicare and other public programs, of whether reimbursement is justified. Such an office could also help determine when government support is warranted for orphan technologies, which have potential to cure diseases that afflict relatively small numbers of people.

In 1984, Congress took a step in this direction by giving the National Center for Health Services Research statutory responsibility for health care technology assessment and for advising the Secretary of Health and Human Services whether federally financed programs should reimburse for use of specific technologies. In addition, Congress for the first time required that extensions of reimbursement to new medical procedures take into account cost-effectiveness and limits of appropriate use, as well as safety and efficacy. Unfortunately, as is too often the case, Congress has not backed up its good intentions with sufficient funds to support a serious technology assessment effort.

The Food and Drug Administration should conduct research, on a continuing basis, on the effectiveness of drugs that are on the market, and periodically publish its findings. Many of these drugs are ineffective and indiscriminately prescribed by doctors who know far less about them than pharmaceutical company hawkers. The cost savings could be significant. The FDA can also review new drug applications much more promptly.

Far more research must be devoted to addiction. The economic cost of addiction is at least $200 billion in health care, disability payments, lost productivity, accidents, crime; the cost in health care alone approaches $50 billion. Yet we devote less than $150 million out of a research budget of $11 billion to the problem. Despite the widespread diseases alcoholism and alcohol abuse cause, they are near the bottom of the list in private research support: alcoholism gets 30 cents per victim, while cancer gets $66, cystic fibrosis $131, and muscular dystrophy $173.

We should establish a National Institute of Addiction in the National Institutes of Health. Such an institute would combine the research work of the National Institutes of Drug Abuse and of Alcohol Abuse and Alcoholism, and conduct research on all substance abuse and multiple addiction, including cigarette smoking. Addiction is a problem as defiantly resistant to solution as is cancer; it is difficult to get our best minds persistently concentrated on preventing and treating addiction, in part because the problem is so infernally complex, and in part because the level and commitment of funds for research have been erratic. Combining the research work of the alcohol and drug abuse institutes and creating one for all addiction would help generate a steady stream of money for research, make clear our national commitment, and attract more of our best minds to the effort.

We must direct greater research efforts to health promotion and disease prevention for the elderly and for adolescents. We should mount a massive effort to attack problems like memory loss, disorientation, and incontinence, which inhibit the ability of the elderly to live independently or with modest help at home. Many habits that persist for a lifetime are started in the adolescent years; we can learn more about how to instill the healthy ones, and how to resist the pull of some adolescents to addiction.

THE MONEY CHANGERS

The Blues, Cross and Shield, and the health insurance companies, stock and mutual, have for decades viewed themselves as representatives of the health care industry. Large corporate purchasers have begun to turn this attitude around. By private initiative, tradition, and law, the money changers should understand that their pledge of allegiance goes to the people who pay their bills: individual patients, corporations, and unions. Only then will these insurers become tough bargainers with health providers, prudent purchasers of medical care, and junkyard watchdogs over physician and hospital practices, alert for waste, overutilization, and abuse.

By every method possible, we must render the Blues and commercial health insurers more responsible to the patients and those paying the bills. Corporations buying services from the Blues and private insurers should insist on the same degree of responsiveness that they demand from other suppliers. Purchasers of health insurance should insist upon tight contractual relationships that make clear the legal liability of insurers that do not fulfill their responsibilities or fail to erect screens to prevent payments for unnecessary medical procedures.

The Blues and commercial insurers are beginning to question inefficient practices of hospitals. They should confront physicians as well, to ask those who charge twice as much or more for the same services why they do so, and to promote a more sensible balance in payments to specialists, general surgeons, and family physicians, by better relating fees to skill, complexity of medical procedure, and costs. They should establish professional screens and cost-benefit standards for all physician care. They should seek out the most efficient providers of medical services.

Our health insurance companies should reorient their targets of insurance. Medical services follow reimbursement dollars the way an alley cat hunts fish in the garbage. Our insurance patterns should be shifted, providing better coverage for preventive care and health promotion—for example, offering fuller reimbursement for periodic checkups than for treatments of marginal benefit to the patient. HMO coverage should be offered as one option by most, if not all, insurers. Our system has been so lopsidedly tilted toward hospital care that it has inhibited shifting many medical procedures out of the hospital and into the doctor's office. Most preadmission testing and all sorts of minor surgery would already have been moved to physicians' offices if medical insurance paid the bill for work there to the extent it has paid for the same work in far more expensive hospital settings.

Of particular importance can be a willingness to provide health insurance coverage for care at home and in hospices and nursing homes. Since 1983 Medicare has covered some such care. But most private plans don't cover any, while they pay through the nose for high-technology deaths in hospital intensive care units. Why not cover care at home or in a hospice, where an individual with terminal illness can die in dignity, with much of the pain relieved, holding the hands of his loved ones, rather than hooked to tubes and plastic and metal machines? Commercial insurers and the Blues can help lead the way to seeking imaginative financial solutions to cover home health and nursing home care.

BIG BUSINESS AT THE HOSPITAL BED
AND IN THE DOCTOR'S OFFICE

The injection of traditional business principles—competition, price shopping, tough negotiating—into the health care arena has been salutary. Corporate America is beginning to get more value for its health care dollars. For-profit health care providers on the other side of the table are also introducing some beneficial competition and sophisticated management.

There is a profound public interest in how health care providers pursue profits. The great crash of 1929 showed us that the banking and securities industries involved a public trust that required public oversight. Similarly, the excesses of steel, railroad, and oil industries sparked antitrust laws to help big competitors resist the urge to monopolize. The public's stake in health care is perhaps greater than its stake in any other economic enterprise—analogous to the need to maintain rigorous safety standards in the airline industry, but infinitely more complex, immediate, and dynamic, and intimately touching far more people.

The profit motive cannot be permitted to shortchange quality of care or curtail access to needed medical services. Special precautions are needed as the big-money men move into the health care system in large, integrated corporate structures. The rise of for-profit hospital chains, and their ventures of vertical integration with suppliers of medical products, can't be viewed only in an economic dimension. The temptation to excessive use of medical devices—drugs and X-rays, for example—increases in a hospital that supplies itself. It is essential to develop standards to protect the patient from unnecessarily risky medical care and unjustified costs. In the first instance, competition and DRG systems will help, but they alone are not enough.

The unique nature of health care requires that high ethical and medical standards be set. Corporate and government purchasers of care can use their leverage to protect their patients, but the introduction of the profit motive requires a special vigilance. Big business brings its own set of values to the hospital bedside and the doctor-patient relationship. We must adopt rules for the profiters to live by as they take over more of the health industry, so that our nation can get the most of their efficiency, maintain the highest professional standards, and ensure that they take their fair share of Medicaid and poor patients. Devising such rules deserves top priority of medical societies, federal, state, and local government, and each of us as citizens.

Developing these standards merits immediate attention, for

here the forces of change have a special electricity. Corporate purchasers, realizing that careful shopping for health care will produce a heftier bottom line, are becoming aggressive proponents of cost-saving techniques—HMOs, second surgical opinions, preadmission review, outpatient testing, hospital DRGs, and others—and they want fast results. So does a deficit-conscious government. In 1985, as soon as the Blues offered Chrysler Corporation lower rates for its salaried employees than the HMOs offered, Chrysler asked the HMOs to come in below the Blues.

Providers of health care, scrambling in this newly sophisticated and tough-minded market, are reorganizing rapidly to compete for the health care dollars of business and government. The financing and the delivery of health care are becoming integrated, led by the for-profit chains. Emerging health care conglomerates hope to create a guaranteed clientele for their hospital beds and at the same time control costs and utilization. These new health conglomerates enjoy a number of competitive advantages over single-purpose hospital or insurance companies. As insurance companies, they have much greater leverage on the claims they will face because they control the providers—their own hospitals and clinics. As hospitals and clinics, they can operate at efficient capacities by providing incentives in their insurance plans to encourage patients to go to them.

Humana, Hospital Corporation of America, and other hospital chains boosted enrollment in their one-year-old health insurance programs to more than 1 million subscribers in 1985. Like other health conglomerates, Humana and HCA offer substantial discounts for patients who use their hospitals and physicians, and higher copayments and deductibles for those who use others.

With companies soliciting bids from all comers, these new health conglomerates are sparking a change in the traditional ways of business of Blue Cross/Blue Shield, the commercial insurers, the HMOs, and the voluntary hospitals. In 1985 Prudential Insurance Company started developing sixty managed health care programs of its own—particularly tuned to reduce unnecessary hospital use—throughout the country, including a joint venture with Group Health, Incorporated, one of Minneapolis's largest and oldest HMOs. Seeking to secure its share of this rapidly growing market, the 450-member Voluntary Hospitals of America, an association of nonprofit hospitals, in 1985 announced a joint venture with Aetna Life and Casualty Company to offer health insurance and care through its member hospitals, with a prediction of 5 million to 10 million subscribers by 1990. And the Blues scrambled to set up one hundred of their own HMOs and preferred providers.

Whether the trend toward consolidation will result, as some have predicted, in ten to fifteen corporations delivering most medical care in the United States, it is clear that bare-knuckled competition will increase and that a significant degree of consolidation is likely. As a nation, we will pay dearly if we do not get the rules of the road in place to oblige the new conglomerates—for-profit and nonprofit alike—to respect the special nature of health care and to provide quality care to all Americans.

THE STATES AND CITIES

State and local governments, the strong grass roots of governing America, have crucial roles to play in the health care revolution.

First, they should open up much of the practice of medicine to paraprofessionals, such as properly educated nurses, and ease monopolistic and unduly restrictive laws. Passed with the best of intentions to protect consumers, these laws have been perpetuated and perverted to hurt them by keeping fees high. Too often, they shelter the economic interest of doctors by preserving medical monopolies and prohibiting qualified paraprofessionals from performing procedures, like routine examinations, cleaning and stitching minor injuries, and treating sprains, minor colds, flus, and stomach disorders. On January 1, 1985, the nation's hospital accreditation body abandoned its requirement that hospital "medical staffs" be limited to doctors, thus opening them up to nurse-midwives, psychologists, and a host of other practitioners. The states can move on a much broader scale.

Dentists have evidenced far more flexibility than doctors in using paraprofessionals. But even here, state laws with broad definitions of dentistry that can be performed by dentists only should be changed. A manager of the Reynolds dental HMO in Winston-Salem, North Carolina, told me that the major obstacles to further cost reduction—with no loss in quality of care—were state laws restricting to dentists performance of a host of procedures that paradentals and technicians could easily do. States (and the federal government) can also help open up the practice of both dentistry and medicine by permitting direct reimbursement for paraprofessional services.

Second, state and local laws should do their part to encourage publication of charges and other health care information. They should require doctors, dentists, hospitals, and all other health providers to furnish full information about charges, in advance, to all patients, and make available at offices, in waiting rooms of doctors and hospitals and clinics, lists of medical procedures performed and the complete charges for these procedures. Patients, particularly elderly ones, who are often easily confused, should be told, up front, whether the doctor or other medical service provider intends to charge them more than their insurance covers.

Third, states should move to eliminate malpractice abuses. In reality, the cost of malpractice insurance is paid not by doctors and hospitals but by all of us as taxpayers and patients, and in 1984 it came close to $4 billion of our health care bill.

In New York the situation came to a head in 1985 when State Insurance Superintendent James Corcoran okayed a 52 percent increase in malpractice insurance for doctors, calling the hike "ridiculous" even as he announced it. New York physicians, who paid $264 million in malpractice insurance in 1984, were told they'd have to pay an additional $158 million in 1985—a total of $422 million. A typical Long Island obstetrician's annual cost for malpractice coverage was scheduled to jump from $54,282 to $82,500; a neurosurgeon's from $66,468 to $101,000; that of a pediatrician providing children with routine, family care, from $10,689 to $16,200.

In response, Governor Mario Cuomo and the state legislature fashioned emergency legislation to moderate the increases. The new law, passed in June 1985, reduces lawyers' contingency fees, requires juries to stretch large awards over periods up to ten years, penalizes lawyers and plaintiffs who bring frivolous suits, and sets up optional arbitration procedures. The law also directs hospitals to review doctors' credentials more carefully and to collect systematically information on adverse outcomes; it orders doctors to disclose prior malpractice judgments against them when they apply for hospital privileges. Based on the law, Insurance Superintendent Corcoran cut the malpractice insurance increases by 15 percent. Even with the cut, the biggest single component of cost in many Long Island doctors' bills is not their nurses, rent, or amortization of office equipment. It's the cost of medical malpractice insurance.

To achieve fundamental reform, states must get medical malpractice out of the courtroom and into the administrative law arena, with limits on the amount of recovery. Such limits would provide modest payment for pain and suffering, but largely be linked to costs of health care, rehabilitation, and replacing reasonable loss of income due to inability to work. In cases of wrongful death caused by malpractice, there would be limits related to the reasonable loss of income to the surviving spouse or children. There are ample analogies in workers' compensation and arbitration procedures that can be adapted to this crisis. Contingent legal fees should also be reduced. In 1985, the United States Supreme Court let stand California court decisions upholding a state law with a $250,000 limit on noneconomic malpractice awards and a sharply reduced scale for contingent legal fees.

Malpractice itself needs to be redefined. Doctors should be held to reasonable standards of care. States should set standards that are reasonable locally, to the hospital, doctor, or clinic where the patient goes, and not impose impossible-dream standards on every doctor and hospital in America. The tests doctors truly need to diagnose and treat their patients should be sufficient for their lawyers to prevail in the courtroom.

The skyrocketing costs of malpractice insurance are due in part to the inability of the medical profession and government watchdogs to keep incompetent physicians out of the clinic and the operating room. For doctors, reform of malpractice laws begins at home, with reform of their own medical discipline systems.

Professional medical disciplinary systems are too often not doing their job. In 1984 state medical boards in Nevada, Utah, Oregon, and Mississippi each disciplined more than one physician out of every hundred. But boards in New York, Massachusetts, Nebraska, Hawaii, and the District of Columbia disciplined less than one per thousand. Delaware and Alaska took no actions at all.

State medical boards frequently lack the resources and funding to monitor and investigate problem doctors. Few hospitals perform extensive background checks on physicians to whom they grant privileges, or keep an eye on their performance. Hospitals and doctors are reluctant to discipline or bring charges against their employees or colleagues. When physicians are disciplined, the process for alerting other states is haphazard. Too often, an incompetent physician is permitted to move quietly on to another state or hospital.

Because states and physicians have not adequately policed the medical profession, malpractice litigation represents one of the few formal mechanisms to combat negligent medicine. But in a system that allows physicians with malpractice records simply to take their black bags to a new state or hospital, isolated lawsuits are unlikely to serve as effective deterrents. Nor do they protect the victims of malpractice. Patricia Danzon, a professor at Duke University's Center for Health Policy, estimates that for every one hundred persons injured from malpractice, only ten file claims and only about four receive compensation through court action.

The states must put in place timely and tough license revocation procedures and effective methods to identify and weed out physicians and other providers who pose a threat to the public. Medicare peer review organizations should be required to report problem hospitals and doctors to state licensing boards. Since most malpractice cases arise from hospital stays, states should consider making hospitals liable for actions of doctors in their wards and operating rooms. This would motivate hospitals carefully to screen physicians and keep track of their on-the-job performance.

Changes in state laws relating to physician monopolization of medicine and malpractice are keys to putting an end to medical featherbedding. It is an article of economic faith that featherbedding brought down the American railroads, and that unreasonable work rules make it far more expensive to do everything from delivering mail to manufacturing cars and television sets.

State and local laws, and their support of medical society work rules, unrealistic medical malpractice standards, and ineffective medical discipline systems, have generated a level of medical featherbedding and unreasonable practices as outrageous as any experienced by our railroads. For example, physicians conduct scores of medically unwarranted tests—especially on hospital patients with rich insurance coverage—simply to defend themselves against feared lawsuits. Such practices would not be tolerated in a competitive environment without artificial monopolies and with a rational legal system defining what constitutes negligence and reasonable compensation for injury.

UNCLE SAM'S MEDICAL SYSTEMS

The federal government has got to get its fragmented house in order. Medicare and Medicaid, the Veterans Administration health care system, and, to the fullest measure consistent with wartime needs, the Defense Department's as well, should all be under the same authority. All should use an expanded and refined DRG system.

The complexities of health care, the costly third-party reimbursement systems, and the political and financial power of the doctors, hospitals, and drug and medical equipment corporations drive most government policymakers who touch the system, conservative or liberal, toward price and wage controls. That's where Richard Nixon ended up and where Jimmy Carter tried to get. Even the Reagan administration, out of desperation, froze doctors' Medicare fees. But federal wage and price controls should be regarded as temporary expedients.

My own experience leads me to conclude that lasting solutions to cost problems do not lie in wage and price controls on doctors, hospitals, and other providers. They will be found in changing the financial incentives—how doctors and hospitals are paid, and how patients get their bills paid. The cost-plus, fee-for-service, third-party reimbursement system, with unlimited choice and little or no financial pain for the patient and no incentives to efficiency for the providers, should be scrapped. The federal government can help lead the way by strengthening its DRG system, adopting a fee-for-illness payment system for doctors, and attending to restructuring the system, rather than playing the health care cost shell game.

Federal payment programs can also take a lead in reorienting care to the least expensive necessary. They can encourage elderly patients to stay out of hospitals and nursing homes by providing tax deductions for the cost of caring for those seventy-five and over at homes of children or grandchildren, and by reimbursing the elderly themselves for the cost of health aides. Some states, including Arizona, Oregon, and Idaho, have begun to move in this direction.

The federal government should also sharply increase the tax levied on cigarettes and alcohol (the states can get into this act, too). In 1984, in one of its crudest acts of public policy and money politics, Congress in the very same bill increased the amount the elderly had to pay for Medicare benefits and left in place a scheduled 50 percent cut in the tax on cigarettes. In view of the fact that smoking is perhaps the largest single contributor to high-ticket illnesses like cancer and heart disease, the tax on cigarettes should be increased sharply—at least doubled and ideally quadrupled—to discourage smoking and require the tobacco companies to pay a far greater share of the health care costs they impose on America. The American Lung Association reported that when the cigarette tax was raised from 8 cents to 16 cents a pack in 1983, teenage smoking dropped 14 percent. The federal excise tax exemption for smokeless tobacco, like snuff and chewing tobacco, is unconscionable; such tobacco should be as heavily taxed as cigarettes to help stem its rapidly growing use, especially among teenagers and even younger children.

Similarly, taxes on alcohol—beer, wine, and liquor—should be hiked. In real values, since 1951, when Congress set the federal excise tax on liquor at $10.50 per 100-proof gallon—a tax that applied through 1984—the world has changed. A pair of shoes that cost $10.50 in 1951 cost more than $30.00 in 1984; a train ride that cost $10.50 in 1951 cost $45.00 in 1984; a visit to a doctor's office that cost $10.50 in 1951 cost $70.00 in 1984. Between 1960 and 1985, the real price to the consumer of a bottle of hard liquor dropped almost 60 percent; of beer, more than 30 percent; of wine, about 30 percent. Congress moved the tax on liquor to $12.50 per gallon in 1985. If the tax had been raised to reflect inflation, it would have been set at $40.

The government could play an even more effective role in reducing the number of doctors and getting more medical school graduates into rural areas and inner city ghettos. Federal and state governments could target grants to medical schools that reduce enrollments, particularly for specialists, or agree to train more primary care physicians. It could provide tuition grants only to students who agree to spend at least two (perhaps three) years on assignment in the National Health Service Corps, which should be revitalized to achieve the goal of providing medical services in remote areas and inner cities. No medical school in America can survive without federal aid. As Medicare and private insurers tighten their belts, medical schools face a tough financial crunch, and federal aid to medical schools becomes even more important. That aid should be sufficient to maintain the high quality of our schools and teaching hospitals, but it should be used to get them to train our doctors to participate in a new health care system.

The federal government can also do better in dealing with abuses in the system, and there are plenty of them. Because millions of transactions are involved, it has been difficult to audit health care abuses by doctors and pharmacists, but we have the technology to do so. Computer policing should be widely used by governments (as well as by private insurers and the Blues).

Government actions can have far-reaching influence on the shape of the health care revolution. But the economic stakes are so high, the entrenched interests so powerful, and money has become such an integral and sinister element of legislative politics that we should place our bets for innovative and imaginative solutions more heavily on the private sector than on federal or state government.

CORPORATE AMERICA

Big business can put pressure on doctors and hospitals to reform without the political inhibitions that have made it so difficult for government to act effectively. Corporate mangers don't need political contributions from medical and hospital associations. Rather, the doctors, dentists, and hospitals need the paying customers of American medicine. The difference shows in the speed of change when top executives decide to move on health care costs, in contrast to the erratic pace of government actions.

Aroused American businessmen are the critical catalysts we need to provide a variety of effective answers to the problems of escalating health care costs. Their actions in the early 1980s indicate that even the Rip Van Winkles with the longest beards are waking up to the heavy price of health care and moving to free themselves from costs over which they have little control.

Chrysler, the other automobile companies, and other corporations with high concentrations of employees in a single area can quickly get a handle on their costs. They have the leverage to get utilization data on their insured employees out of the Blues or commercial insurers; they can negotiate with doctors and hospitals to establish preferred providers and direct contracts for care at prearranged prices; they can establish their own health maintenance organizations; they can contract with the federal government to provide Medicare benefits to retirees at a fixed cost that will reward their efficiency.

Smaller employers, or branches of larger companies with a small number of employees in an area, can band together to amass the necessary leverage to set up the same kinds of delivery systems. Since 1980 more than 150 such coalitions have been formed. In California, such a group got legislation passed to permit preferred provider arrangements without violating price discrimination or antitrust laws. In St. Louis, a coalition set up a utilization review process that cut costs by $5 million in the first year. In other cities, employers have combined to get better insurance rates and to press hospitals to post their daily rates and prices for medical procedures.

Business is starting to move. Remarkably, the force in the private industrial community that is most reluctant to give up the status quo is big labor. Too many union negotiators find themselves standing arm in arm with fee-for-service doctors and cost-based hospitals, by and large opposing change because they think their dwindling memberships want it that way. The UAW is beginning to evidence more flexibility, particularly in their 1984 Rockwell settlement and their 1985 auto contracts. But most unions want to keep the plans they have; they oppose deductibles and copayments, even as incentives to get employees to join less costly HMOs and preferred providers where first-dollar coverage would be provided. Some union negotiators talk about unlimited freedom of choice with no payment by employees as though the principle were enshrined in the U.S. Constitution.

Business can also have a major impact in health promotion and disease prevention—by encouraging exercise and providing opportunities for it, by instituting antismoking campaigns and early detection and assistance programs for alcohol and drug abusers. Johnson and Johnson's Live for Life program has demonstrated the potential savings here. Tenneco Incorporated reported that claims for women employees who exercised in 1984 averaged less than half the amounts of those filed by women employees who didn't exercise. Shell Oil found its wellness program cost-effective. Industry can also press the Blues and commercial insurers to tilt coverage toward the least expensive treatment rather than the hospital. It can get coverage of home health, nursing home, and hospice care for the elderly. In short, the genius of American business is critical in shaping the American health care revolution. Business can provide the financial incentives to which we know the hospitals and doctors will respond.

A NEW HEALTHY AMERICA COMPACT

We need a new social compact to govern America's health care system, and goals to measure our progress.

No compassionate society can deny the right of its citizens to the health care they need. We in America have done that for too long. We are the only industrial society of Western (and Far Eastern) civilization that does not recognize such a right. We have quarreled endlessly about national health plans, socialized medicine, freedom of choice. We don't need a national health plan to make adequate health care a right, available to every American. We need to get costs under control, and we need an imaginative and aggressive private sector, a government that stops playing a shell game with health care costs, and a people with the compassion to take care of the poor, the old, and the unemployed.

First, let's recognize the best of our health care system and build on it. Most Americans, about 140 million out of our population of 235 million, have some health care coverage through their employment relationship. Let's simply require that each employer subject to the minimum wage law assure its employees of a minimum level of health care: physician treatment, hospitalization, preventive services for the employee and his or her family. The employer could provide that care however it wished: through insurance, a health maintenance organization, preferred provider contracts, or directly. But the employer would have to pay only the cost of such coverage under the least expensive plan. Other plans could of course be offered. But if the employer did not choose to pay the extra expense, the employee would have to pay the difference. This would encourage competition in the marketplace, and press employers and workers to seek the best plan at the lowest cost. For the small employers and the self-employed, a government corporation should be set up to provide competitive group rates and access to health maintenance organizations and preferred providers. All employers would of course remain free to provide greater health care benefits, and unions would have the right to bargain for them.

Second, for the poor, the elderly, and the temporarily unemployed, government should provide health care coverage. If we want to get the full benefits from a reoriented, truly competitive health care system, it is imperative for government to fulfill this responsibility. As corporate and other big buyers of health care press providers to be more efficient, there will be little maneuvering room to provide Robin Hood care for the needy. Competitive forces signal an end even to well-intentioned cost shifting to pay for the poor, the elderly, and the unemployed by charging the well-insured more for physicians' services and hospitalization.

Yet it is corporate America's aggressive pursuit of lower-cost quality health care that holds the best hope of getting the system to the level of efficiency needed to provide care for all at a reasonable cost. Social justice requires us to provide health care to the poor, the elderly, and the unemployed. In addition, common-sense self-interest encourages us to provide such care for the elderly so that our corporations are not overburdened with the costs of health care for retirees, costs that make it difficult to compete in world markets where virtually all other industrial nations' governments provide such coverage. There are about 33 million Americans without health insurance coverage; no other industrial nation has such a gap. With America's affluence, no excuse for this offense to social justice remains.

We should set cost-containment goals, aiming to provide care for our people at a far lower cost than is now projected. Instead of approaching $700 billion in health care costs by 1990 and topping $1 trillion in 1995, we should be a healthier people for a total bill of $600 billion in 1990 and $800 billion in 1995. That's still about 10.5 percent of our gross national product, but it's a savings of almost $100 billion in 1990 and $250 billion in 1995.

Most important, we must set goals for a Healthy America compact. As virtually my last act as Secretary of Health, Education, and Welfare, on July 26, 1979, I issued the first (and only) Surgeon General's Report on Health Promotion and Disease Prevention. We set goals that can still be achieved by 1990 if all of us work at it.

Here are some new goals for the year 2000:

Infant Mortality: We are at 10.6 deaths per 1,000, well on our way to the 1990 goal of 9.0 per 1,000. The rate of decline has slowed, but with a concerted effort, we can make that goal. Let's assume we reach the 1990 mark on time and set as our goal for the year 2000 reducing infant mortality by an additional 25 percent— to 6.75 deaths per 1,000. Japan is currently at 7 per 1,000 and

Holland at 8 per 1,000. A major factor will be cutting the infant mortality rate among blacks, which is still almost double the rate for white infants.

Children one to fourteen: We have almost achieved the 1990 goal of 34 deaths per 100,000. Let's assume we reach 30 per 100,000 by 1990. Another 20 percent reduction is a reasonable goal. That would bring us to 24 per 100,000 in the year 2000.

Adolescents and young adults, aged fifteen to twenty-four: We are close to the 1990 goal of 93 deaths per 100,000—the current rate is 96 per 100,000. It is reasonable to expect that we will reach 90 per 100,000 in 1990. A further reduction of 25 percent seems possible by the year 2000, for a rate of 68 per 100,000. The big factors here are auto accidents, especially for white males, and homicides, especially for black males.

Adults, aged twenty-five to sixty-four: At 454 deaths per 100,000, we are on course for the 1990 goals of 400 per 100,000. Aiming for another 25 percent reduction by 2000 would give the nation a goal of 300 per 100,000.

For those sixty-five and older: The 1990 goal is a 20 percent reduction in the average days of illness per year, and a significant improvement in mobility and self-sufficiency. This has been a difficult and somewhat unpredictable measure as more people live longer. The rate of restricted-activity days per year went from 36.5 in 1977 up to 39.9 in 1981, and then down to 31.6 in 1982. Assuming that this measure has validity, we should press to reach 28 days by 1990, then reduce it to 23 days by 2000. The central point is to get our energies concentrated on increased self-sufficiency and mobility for the elderly over seventy-five.

Government can help establish the consensus and be a catalyst. Congress, as our representative national voice, might even pass a Healthy America Act, committing our nation to health promotion and disease prevention, authorizing the publication of Healthy America goals, and providing some seed money to help get us all aware of them.

But government alone can't achieve these goals. The private sector should lead this effort, and everyone must join in if it is to work. We need widespread publicity in the media, the workplace, schools, and union halls. Each state and community should measure itself against the goals. Each individual should strive to take better care of himself or herself.

The central fact about health care and costs in America is that we can do something about them. We can't create heaven on earth, but we have the capacity to provide quality care for all at reasonable cost. We can shape a competitive system of excellence, and motivate doctors and hospitals to provide less expensive care and patients to stay healthy. We have the moral depth and Judeo-Christian base to face the bewildering ethical issues our scientists pose with their ingenious biomedical and technological inventions and manipulations.

Our fate is in our hands. The uncertainties are not in knowing what to do, not in science, not in economics. The uncertainties lie in our ability to discipline ourselves and our individual and collective wills to act with courage and compassion in a host of forums, from the Congress, state legislatures, city halls, school boards, hospital and corporate boardrooms, and union halls to doctors' offices and our own homes.

Who lives? Who dies? Who pays?

That's up to us.

Afterword

Since this book was first published, the American Health Care Revolution it describes has assumed hurricane force.

The winds of convulsive change continue to buffet the business of health care. Miracle drugs, electronics, lasers and nuclear scanners are radically reshaping the landscape of diagnosis, disease and care. Scientific and pharmaceutical discoveries are so revolutionizing the treatment of coronary heart disease that many cardiac surgeons may soon find their specialty as obsolete as picking cotton by hand. Each dawn seems to bring yet another spectacular advance, and just over the horizon we can see a world of biotechnology beyond the imagination of Steven Spielberg. At the eye of the storm, a medical alphabet of HMOs, PPOs, IPAs (Independent Practice Associations) and INC.s scramble with fee-for-service physicians and voluntary hospitals for a piece of the health care action that will top 620 billion dollars in 1989.

But the more everything keeps changing, the more one thing remains the same: health care costs keep rocketing.

- Health insurance premiums jumped an average of some 25 percent in 1988 and about the same amount again in 1989, with some hikes a dizzying 70 percent each of those years.
- One year into the 1990s, Americans will spend 2 billion dollars *each day* on health care.
- In 1989, we're spending 85 billion dollars for Medicare and 235 billion dollars for Social Security. Just after the year 2000, we'll

spend more on Medicare than on Social Security—600 billion dollars on Medicare, 595 billion dollars on Social Security.

Research completed since this book was first published has confirmed its estimate that at least 25 percent of the money we spend on health care is wasted. That's more than $150 billion in 1989—some $3 billion a week! In a nation where 37 million citizens do not have access to basic health insurance or care, in a Congress that agonizes over annual deficit reductions of far less than that amount, in an era of increasing international competitive pressure on large corporations and unions to cut costs, such profligacy is unconscionable.

Thanks to years of work by Medicare and Rand Corporation professionals and others like Dr. John Wennberg at Dartmouth, we know that billions of the dollars we spend on many medical and surgical procedures—such as coronary bypasses, cesarean sections, pacemakers, tonsillectomies and hysterectomies—have little or no impact on the health of thousands of the patients subjected to them.

Medical experts now believe that 26 percent of the coronary angiographies, 28 percent of the endoscopies of the upper gastrointestinal tract, and 64 percent of the carotid endarterectomies performed are of no or uncertain value. Even in circumstances in which most doctors agree that particular treatments are warranted, there are still enormous variations—some more than tenfold—in the rates at which people in different places are subjected to risky and expensive surgical procedures with no apparent relation to their health.

We don't need to spend lots more money on health care. We already spend more than enough to provide care for all our people, including those without health insurance, if only we would spend it wisely.

The pressing task for physicians and hospital administrators is to find out what works and what doesn't—in short, to determine what quality care is. It's time for a rigorous effort to establish which procedures produce beneficial outcomes under what conditions and to eliminate stark instances of overutilization such as those cited above. Costs aside, subjecting patients to high-risk surgical procedures that have little or no likelihood of affecting their health raises profound ethical questions.

The pursuit of quality care need not involve cookie-cutter medicine or stifle the creativity that has made American medicine the envy of the world. And in areas where standards can be established they can serve as a safe haven for doctors, protecting them from unjustified malpractice claims.

If the professionals procrastinate, government and other big buyers of health care will act. Surging costs will spur these purchasers to insist that they pay only for procedures that can be shown to affect the medical outcome.

Defining quality health care will not be easy. We are trying to determine the best way to treat a patient, judge the competence of doctors, nurses and lab technicians, and quantify a number of intangibles. But computers make it possible to measure outcomes of medical procedures by analyzing rates of relapse, readmission, surgical rupture and infection, length of hospital stays, length of recovery time, time away from work, death rates and other data.

The need for a sea change in patient and physician attitudes has become increasingly clear. Patients must not only recognize their responsibility to take care of themselves. A fundamental cultural shift of patient expectations about health care and physician conduct is essential. Presently, in most cases of uncertainty about the value of a medical procedure, the physician's approach is: unless a procedure has been shown to be ineffective, try it. Patients in discomfort usually agree.

Perhaps physicians and patients should adopt a different attitude: unless the procedure has been proven effective, don't use it.

There is ample precedent for doctors and surgeons to make this cultural shift. The FDA requires that drugs be proven safe and effective before they can be marketed. Drug companies spend millions of dollars supporting years of study to demonstrate the safety and benefits of their products. Yet most medical and surgical procedures—which account for far more risk and most health care spending—are subjected to far less scrutiny before they are adopted. A key element of encouraging this cultural shift is to pay doctors to *talk* to their patients, and for patients to accept the fact that fees for that service are often far better spent than to pay doctors only to *do* something to them.

A dramatic reordering of our research priorities is even more urgent than when this book was first published. Big medical research bucks must be devoted to our two largest health care problems: aging and addiction.

As people live longer, the length of time during which they need help in the tasks of daily living increases. The astronomical cost of confronting this dependence has sent tremors through Congress and state capitols, and has drained the savings and psyches of far more American families than catastrophic illness.

Most nursing-home residents and millions of the elderly living at home need help with the basic activities of living—bathing, dressing, using the toilet, and eating. Of the 1.3 million nursing-home residents, almost two thirds suffer from dementia, mental disorientation, or loss of memory. Most suffer from difficulties in walking, often due to rheumatism, arthritis and, particularly for the 90 percent of women over 75 who suffer from osteoporosis, disabling injuries due to falls.

We need a massive effort—a Project Independence for Older Americans—to reduce and, for many of the elderly, eliminate the chief threats to their independence. A Project Independence research program should focus on at least three areas: incontinence, memory loss and immobility.

Independence is what the elderly want most. Is there any son or daughter who would rather spend money to keep parents in a nursing home than to keep them living independently? The more independent the elderly are, the less expensive nursing and institutional care they require. The payoff of Project Independence for Older Americans could be enormous: Each reduction of one month in the average period of dependence means a saving of up to $4 billion in health care and custodial costs.

If we're serious about America's drug crisis, it will take more than public education and harsher penalties. We must learn why it's so hard to say no—and how to make it easier. The persistent spread of substance abuse and addiction and their fallouts in disease, injury and teenage pregnancy have confirmed the need for a national institute of addiction, as part of the National Institutes of Health, to conduct research on all substance abuse including smoking, alcohol and pills, as well as marijuana, cocaine, crack and heroin.

Politicians, as well as patients and physicians, need to exercise some self-discipline. A cynical cycle of legislatively induced health care inflation too often marks the actions of Congress. Congress adds new benefits in an inefficient and needlessly expensive way (as it has done with the catastrophic care bill, achieving a highly desirable end through financially reckless means); Congress grossly underestimates the cost of the benefits; as the true price tag becomes apparent to the taxpayers, Congress lashes out at the doctors, hospitals and pharmaceutical companies for inefficiency and price gouging and at the executive branch (of whatever party) for lax administration and corruptly cozying up to health care providers. Rarely does Congress examine, much less accept, its own culpability in the way it drafted the legislation in the first place.

I've come to visualize our health care system as a mountain-climbing team struggling to scale an extremely steep cliff en route to a Mount Everest of quality care for all. The lead climbers are our spectacular scientific genius and superb doctors and medical centers. But then come those who have lost their footing. One dangling climber is the hospitals, with their empty beds. Another is technology, swinging loose on the rope, unbridled by considerations of the relationship of cost to benefit. Next come lawyers and judges, dragging the team down with malpractice litigation. Then the enormous load of patient expectations, crying out: "Do something, Doctor, up to the limit of my health insurance—and don't hold me responsible for my own health." Finally comes the politician, pandering to providers, needlessly adding to the cost of care.

Our lead climbers must negotiate this slippery cliff in a blinding snowstorm of uncertainty about which medical and surgical procedures truly affect the medical outcome for patients. In a sense, it's remarkable that our health care system is still scaling the cliff. But it cannot hope to reach the heights of quality care for all unless we get all members of the team to do their share.

The stakes in America's health care revolution are high: living, dying, paying fearful prices, confronting vexing ethical choices and, in the end, the continued viability of America's top-quality medical system. Whether we maintain and enhance that system—and make it available to all our citizens—is a decision that cannot be left solely in the hands of physicians and politicians. It is a decision for all of us—employers and workers, patients and citizens.

Note on Sources

Wherever possible, I have relied on information published by government agencies and by widely recognized sources of health care data, such as the American Hospital Association and the Urban Institute. These sources have been supplemented by numerous conversations with experts in many government agencies and health industry associations, with doctors and hospital administrators, with corporate executives and union officials knowledgeable about health care and its costs, and with independent health policy analysts. Listed below are my principal published sources.

Budget of the United States Government, Fiscal Years 1985 and 1986 (U.S. Office of Management and Budget, Washington, D.C., 1984, 1985); *Caring for the Older Veteran* (Veterans Administration, Washington, D.C., 1984); *Economic Costs to Society of Alcohol and Drug Abuse and Mental Illness: 1980*, Final Report (prepared by Research Triangle Institute for the U.S. Department of Health and Human Services, Research Triangle Park, N.C., 1984); *Federal Policies and the Medical Devices Industry* (U.S. Congress, Office of Technology Assessment, Washington, D.C., 1984); *Fifth Special Report to the U.S. Congress on Alcohol and Health from the Secretary of Health and Human Services* (U.S. Department of Health and Human Services, Washington, D.C., 1983); *Health, United States, 1983* and *Health, United States, 1984* (U.S. Department of Health and Human Services, Washington, D.C., 1983, 1984); *Medicaid and Nursing Home Care: Cost Increases and the Need for Services Are Creating Problems for the*

States and the Elderly (U.S. General Accounting Office, Washington, D.C., 1984); *Medical Education and Societal Needs: A Planning Report for the Health Professions* (National Academy of Sciences, Institute of Medicine, Washington, D.C., 1984); *Medical Technology and the Costs of the Medicare Program* (U.S. Congress, Office of Technology Assessment, Washington, D.C., 1984); *Medicare and the Health Costs of Older Americans: The Extent and Effects of Cost Sharing* (U.S. Senate, Special Committee on Aging, S. Prt. 98-166, Washington, D.C., 1984); *Medicare Benefits and Financing Report of the 1982 Advisory Council on Social Security* (U.S. Department of Health and Human Services, Washington, D.C., 1983); *Medicare: Paying the Physician—History, Issues, and Options* (U.S. Senate, Special Subcommittee on Aging, S. Prt. 98-153, Washington, D.C., 1984); *Proceedings of the Conference on the Future of Medicare* (U.S. House of Representatives, Committee on Ways and Means, Subcommittee on Health, WMCP:98-13, Washington, D.C., 1983); *Projections of the Population of the United States, by Age, Sex, and Race: 1983 to 2080* (Bureau of the Census, U.S. Department of Commerce, Washington, D.C., 1984); *Securing Access to Health Care* (President's Commission for the Study of Ethical Problems in Medicine and Biomedical and Behavioral Research, Washington, D.C., 1983); *Short-Term Evaluation of Medicaid: Selected Issues* (U.S. Department of Health and Human Services, Washington, D.C., 1984); *Semiannual Reports* (Office of the Inspector General, U.S. Department of Health and Human Services, Washington, D.C., October 1979, March 1983, September 1983, March 1984, September 1984); *Statistical Abstract of the United States*, 1984 and 1985 (Bureau of the Census, U.S. Department of Commerce, Washington, D.C., 1983, 1984); *Summary of the 1984 Annual Reports of the Medicare Board of Trustees* and *Summary of the 1985 Annual Reports of the Medicare Board of Trustees* (U.S. Department of Health and Human Services, Washington, D.C., 1984, 1985); *Summary Report of the Graduate Medical Education National Advisory Committee*, Vol. 1 (U.S. Department of Health and Human Services, Washington, D.C., 1980); *Third Report to the President and Congress on the Status of Health Professions Personnel in the United States* (U.S. Department of Health and Human Services, Washington, D.C.,

1982); *U.S. Industrial Outlook 1984* and *U.S. Industrial Outlook 1985* (U.S. Department of Commerce, Washington, D.C., 1984, 1985); *Veterans Administration Health Care: Planning for Future Years* (U.S. Congress, Congressional Budget Office, Washington, D.C., 1984).

Directory of Multihospital Systems, Fourth Edition (American Hospital Publishing, Inc., Chicago, Ill., 1984); *Facts on Long Term Health Care* (American Health Care Association, Washington, D.C., 1984); *1984 Federation of American Hospitals Directory* (Federation of American Hospitals, Washington, D.C., 1984); *Hospital Statistics*, 1983 Edition (American Hospital Association, Chicago, Ill., 1983); *Physician Characteristics and Distribution in the U.S.*, 1982 Edition (American Medical Association, Chicago, Ill., 1983); *SMS Reports* (American Medical Association, Chicago, Ill., 1983, 1984, 1985); *Recent and Proposed Changes in State Medicaid Programs* (Intergovernmental Health Policy Project, George Washington University, Washington, D.C., 1981, 1982, 1983, 1984); *Source Book of Health Insurance Data 1982–1983* and *1984 Update* (Health Insurance Association of America, Washington, D.C., 1983, 1984); *Statistical Profile of the Investor-Owned Hospital Industry, 1982* (Federation of American Hospitals, Washington, D.C., 1984); *Trends* (American Hospital Association, Chicago, Ill., 1983, 1984).

Health and the War on Poverty, by Karen Davis and Cathy Schoen (The Brookings Institution, Washington, D.C., 1978); *Health and Wealth*, by Robert Maxwell (Lexington Books, Lexington, Mass., 1981); *Medicare and the Hospitals*, by Herman Miles Somers and Anne Ramsay Somers (The Brookings Institution, Washington, D.C., 1966); *Medicare: The Politics of Federal Hospital Insurance*, by Judith Feder (Lexington Books, Lexington, Mass., 1977); *The New Health Care for Profit*, edited by Bradford H. Gray (National Academy Press, Washington, D.C., 1983); *The Painful Prescription*, by Henry J. Aaron and William B. Schwartz (The Brookings Institution, Washington, D.C., 1984); *Payer, Provider, Consumer: Industry Confronts Health Care Costs*, by Diana Chapman Walsh and Richard H. Egdahl (Springer-Verlag, New York, N.Y., 1977); *The Politics of Medicare*, by Theodore Marmor (Aldine, New York, N.Y., 1977); *Searching for a Cure*, by Jonas

Morris (PICA Press, New York, N.Y., 1984); *The Reagan Record*, edited by John L. Palmer and Isabel V. Sawhill (The Urban Institute, Ballinger Publishing, Cambridge, Mass., 1984); *The Social Transformation of American Medicine*, by Paul Starr (Basic Books, Inc., New York, N.Y., 1982); *Technology in Hospitals*, by Louise B. Russell (The Brookings Institution, Washington, D.C., 1979); *Who Shall Live*, by Victor Fuchs (Basic Books, Inc., New York, N.Y., 1974); *The X-Ray Information Book*, by Priscilla Laws and the Public Citizen Health Research Group (Farrar, Straus, and Giroux, New York, N.Y., 1974).

Numerous articles published in journals, newspapers, and magazines, including: *Atlantic Monthly; Business and Health; Business Week; Congressional Quarterly; Consumer Exchange* (Blue Cross and Blue Shield Association); *The Economist; Forbes; Health Affairs; Health Care Financing Review; Journal of the American Medical Association; Journal of Medical Education; Milbank Memorial Fund Quarterly; Modern Healthcare; Modern Maturity; National Journal; The New England Journal of Medicine; Newsweek; The New York Daily News; The New York Times; Reader's Digest; Standard and Poor's Industry Surveys; Time; Value Line Investment Survey; The Wall Street Journal; The Washington Monthly; The Washington Post; Washington Report on Health Legislation and Regulation* (McGraw-Hill).

INDEX

About the Author

JOSEPH A. CALIFANO, JR., was born on May 15, 1931, in Brooklyn, New York, where he grew up. He received his Bachelor of Arts degree from the College of the Holy Cross in 1952 and his LL.B. from Harvard Law School in 1955. Mr. Califano then served for three years as a commissioned officer in the office of the Judge Advocate General of the Navy in Washington, D.C. After three years with Governor Thomas Dewey's Wall Street law firm, he joined the Kennedy administration, first as Special Assistant to Defense Department General Counsel Cyrus Vance, and then successively as Special Assistant to the Secretary of the Army, as General Counsel of the Army, and as Secretary of Defense Robert McNamara's Special Assistant and top troubleshooter. President Lyndon Johnson named Mr. Califano his Special Assistant for Domestic Affairs in 1965, a position he held until President Johnson left office on January 20, 1969. During his service in that post, *The New York Times* called him "Deputy President for Domestic Affairs." From 1969 to 1977, Mr. Califano practiced law in Washington, D.C., and served as attorney for *The Washington Post, Newsweek,* and others during the Watergate years. From 1977 to 1979, he was Secretary of Health, Education, and Welfare. Since then he has been practicing law in Washington, D.C. He was Special Counselor to the Governor of the State of New York on Alcoholism and Drug Abuse from 1980 to 1982. Mr. Califano is the author of six previous books (two with Howard Simons, former managing editor of *The Washington Post*) and has written articles for *The New York Times, The Washington Post, Reader's Digest, The New Republic,* and other publications.

Mr. Califano is a member of the board of directors of Primerica Corporation, ADP, Chrysler Corporation, and Health Data Sciences Corporation and a trustee of Georgetown University, New York University, the Urban Institute, the Kaiser Family Foundation, and the Iacocca Foundation. He chairs the Chrysler board's committee on health care, and is recognized as an expert on health care costs and the health care industry, subjects on which he consults and lectures.

He is at present senior partner in the Washington, D.C., office of the law firm of Dewey, Ballantine, Bushby, Palmer and Wood.